THE RADIATION PRO

Drawing on current research Le
nutritional steps can be taken to protect your body
the damaging effects of everyday low-level radiation.

By the same author

ABOUT LAETRILE
A WORLD WITHOUT AIDS (With Simon Martin)
ACUPUNCTURE TREATMENT OF PAIN
AMINO ACIDS IN THERAPY
AN END TO CANCER?
CANDIDA ALBICANS
INSTANT PAIN CONTROL
OSTEOPATHY
SOFT-TISSUE MANIPULATION
THE NEW SELF HELP FOR ATHRITIS
THE NEW SELF HELP FOR FATIGUE
THE NEW SELF HELP FOR HEADACHES AND MIGRAINE
THE NEW SELF HELP FOR HIGH BLOOD PRESSURE
THE NEW SELF HELP FOR VARICOSE VEINS
YOUR COMPLETE STRESS-PROOFING PROGRAMME
YOUR OWN SLIMMING AND HEALTH PROGRAMME

THE RADIATION PROTECTION PLAN

Raise Your Resistance Level to Everyday Radiation

Leon Chaitow
N.D., D.O., M.B.N.O.A.

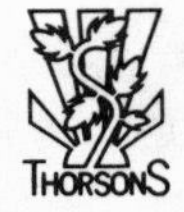

THORSONS PUBLISHING GROUP

First published 1988

British Library Cataloguing in Publication Data

Chaitow, Leon
How to live with low-level radiation:
the nutritional protection plan.
1. Ionizing radiation — Physiological effect
2. Diet therapy
I. Title
612'.014486 QP82.2.I53

ISBN 0-7225-1478-6

Published by Thorsons Publishers Limited, Wellingborough, Northamptonshire, NN8 2RQ, England

Printed in Great Britain by Woolnough Bookbinding Limited, Irthlingborough, Northamptonshire

1 3 5 7 9 10 8 6 4 2

Contents

1. Radiation And Its Dangers

Life on earth has always been exposed to radiation from a variety of earthly and cosmic sources. In a sense the very existence of life as we know it is owed to the effects of radiation, since genetic changes which take place as part of the process of evolution are often triggered by radiation's influence on the DNA, the genetic material of humans, animals and plants or their predecessors.

There are many different types of radiation deriving from a multitude of sources, and the effects these have on different organs and parts of the body vary. In addition to the sudden influx of radiation produced by disasters such as occurred in Russia at Chernobyl, in the USA at Three Mile Island and in the UK at Windscale, we are exposed to other less obvious sources. These include atmospheric residues of nuclear weapon testing; nuclear power station leaks, and wastes; diagnostic and therapeutic use of X-rays in medicine; use of radioactive chemicals in medicine; microwave ovens; the emission waves from radio and television sources; television sets (especially pre-1970 colour sets); computer visual display units; irradiated food; a large number of smoke detectors found in public buildings, shops, hotels etc.; a number of precious stones and metals such as irradiated blue sapphires and old gold; some ceramics and pottery (glazed with uranium oxide); radium found in luminous clocks, and watches (usually old ones); cigarette smoke; cosmic and earth radiation; old houses and buildings constructed of granite, or in which other materials used are radioactive.

Different types of radiation

When we speak of radiation we should be aware of at least two different types. There is what is called ionizing radiation, which derives from radioactive materials, nuclear power stations, nuclear weapon tests and X-ray machines. Cosmic radiation from the sun is also ionizing radiation, as are those rays from the radioactive substances in and on the earth.

The other type of radiation is non-ionizing radiation, such as radio waves, ultra-violet rays, ultra-sound waves, micro-waves, etc. A much greater exposure is required to any of these non-ionizing forms to produce any damage, which would in any case usually show itself immediately rather than as a delayed action result as in the case of ionizing radiation.

When we speak of ionizing radiation we mean that form which breaks down and destroys the cells which comprise our bodies. The ionizing rays which are commonly mentioned include alpha rays, which are easily shielded against, but which are potentially extremely dangerous if they enter the body; beta rays which are a little harder to shield from, requiring at least a thin metal shield to stop them from entering the body, and which cause skin burns and internal damage. There are also the high energy gamma rays which can penetrate the body easily (such as X-rays) and these require a heavy shield such as lead or concrete to stop them penetrating the body.

All three forms of ray are found in nuclear sources and machine-made radiation (X-rays), but only alpha and beta rays are found in cosmic radiation.

What makes the rays different from each other?

There is only one amusing thing about radiation activity and that is the confusion that exists in describing its measurement. If *you* are puzzled after reading the next few paragraphs, do not consider yourself alone, for this is the effect felt by anyone new to this area of science, and even to many who are old hands.

The difference in the physical effects of ionizing radiation depends upon, among other things, the particular wavelength they have (the measured distance from the crest of one wave to the next). The standard unit of measuring wavelengths is the angstrom, named after the Swedish physicist. One angstrom (A) represents one ten millionth of a millimetre, or one tenth of a millimicron. Thus ten angstroms equal one millimicron (written as Greek mu).

After centuries of debate it has been concluded (if anything in physics is ever concluded) that rays consist of enormously large numbers of exceedingly small entities called photons. The photon travels at the speed of light (186,000 miles per second) when in a vacuum, but this slows when it is in contact with a medium such as liquid, or even air, which contains particles of hydrogen etc. Whilst these photons have an actual (if infinitesimally minute) mass, they behave in movement in a wave-like manner. Thus both the size of the photon and the length of the wave which they make in travel, determines the characteristics of a particular form of radiation.

How small?

Cosmic rays which were discovered in 1921 have a wavelength in the air of 0.001 angstrom and a frequency of 3×10^{21}. The frequency of a photon is in proportion to the number of waves which it makes in a second. The smaller the wavelength the greater the frequency, and therefore the greater the energy and potential for destructive force. The very small wavelength photons, with very low angstrom measurements, such as cosmic and gamma rays, have the highest frequencies and do the most damage as they have the greater penetration power.

In 1898 the Curies discovered gamma rays which derive from the substance radium, and which have a wavelength of 1 angstrom (in air) and a frequency of 3×10^{18}. X-rays had been discovered by Roentgen and the scientist Becquerel in 1895, and these have a wavelength of 1.4 to over 100 angstroms and a frequency of 5.9×10^{15}. When we speak of visible rays (colours) we are in the region of thousands of angstrom units.

These introductory technicalities of radiation need not concern you unduly since what matters is that we know the hazards, understand how damage might occur and have a grasp of preventive tactics which can safely be employed.

In any case the actual measurement of radiation as it

reaches, and is absorbed by the body, is where the real confusion begins. The facts of the physical nature of radiation are provided for those who wish to understand the way in which radiation functions.

How do we describe radiation strengths?

The amount of radiation absorbed by the body is usually expressed in terms of rads or rems. These stand for *r*adiation *a*bsorbed *d*ose and *r*adiation dose *e*quivalent in *m*an. It is also sometimes found that the letter R is used to describe the amount of radioactivity which is coming from a particular source (this R stands for roentgen). Rs are the description of radioactivity being emitted by a given source per hour. Smaller doses are measured in milliR or mRs.

The relationship between these measurement symbols is that 1R (roentgen) being emitted from a source (X-ray machine) will deliver 1 rad to the body of a person exposed. The number of rems which the body will absorb will vary though, because rems measure the estimated biologically damaging effect of the dose of radiation. New standard units have been introduced which confuse this reasonably simple description of rads, rems and Rs.

The basic unit expressing the nature of radiation activity is now called a becquerel, which is far smaller than the previously used unit called a curie. One becquerel represents one count per second of radioactivity and is the unit used to measure the amount of radioactivity present in liquids such as milk or water. This is used to describe the content of radioactive iodine in substances.

Rads are also to have their name changed to grays, as are rems which are now called sieverts, although no-one seems to use this term yet. The sievert or rem is the important factor for you and me, since is measures the effect on the body of the dose of radiation. One sievert, incidentally, is the same as 100 rems, and one gray is the same as 100 rads. When it comes to converting a becquerel to a rem the problem becomes more confusing since the type of radiation will influence the number of rems (or sieverts) absorbed, as will other factors.

Thus the effects internally, of absorbed alpha rays will be

higher than those caused by gamma rays, for example. Rem figures will vary as to the type of radiation, and the absorption or otherwise of this. There are many variables which will also influence the degree of damage or otherwise which radiation exposure may cause, and one of the major ones, as we shall see, is nutrition. Other factors include the amount of protective clothing being worn, as well as the distance the person is from the source of radiation.

One source of harmful radiation could be an X-ray machine which is malfunctioning, and therefore emiting undesirable forms of radiation. The major tissue damage which results from excessive radiation exposure derives from a process which is started by the irradiation and which is called *free radical oxidation*.

In addition, the walls of blood vessels and the lining of the digestive tract may be damaged (this being largely the result of free radical activity) causing severe symptoms involving circulation and digestion. The centres for the manufacture of blood may also be damaged, causing subsequent anaemia.

Nutritional methods by which such damage can be controlled or minimized safely, will be discussed in later sections.

Free radicals

It is estimated that in a quart of ordinary air, on a bright sunny day, there will be at least one billion hydroxyl free radicals present, these are the ones that cause the major problems to the body. In city air, polluted with hydrocarbons and heavy metals, the level of dangerous free radicals will be far higher.

We survive this onslaught of dangerous particles by virtue of the presence in our bodies of free radical quenchers, or antioxidants, which prevent the damage to cells from occurring excessively. In a very real sense the process of ageing is the process of free radical damage to tissues.

Tissues, whether they be skin or any other, which are affected by free radical activity, become damaged, and the overall effect is of a less efficient function.

If this occurs in the arteries of the body it represents the onset of atheromatous changes, which end as cardiovascular disease. If it occurs in body cells, and affects the genetic material, then this may be the onset of tumour development. In the case of skin, a loss of elasticity and general wrinkling and toughness takes place; in other words the skin gets older. Radiation damage of the skin will be similar (although far more extreme) to excessive sun bathing, which also triggers free radical activity, which is the reason for the alteration in skin texture and tone when too much sun reaches the body surface.

Rubber that becomes perished or impoverished; metal which rusts, or a peeled potato or apple which changes colour; all these are evidence of oxidation or free radical damage. Bleaching the hair is another example of oxidation in action. But, just as when lemon juice is rubbed onto such a peeled fruit, thus delaying or preventing the colour change; or when a rust-proofing material is used to stop the changes in the metal's state, so in the body it is possible to delay or minimize free radical activity.

The major effect of radiation damage to the body is through such activity, and the proof of the efficacy of a number of anti-free radical strategies has been shown in experimental studies in animals and humans.

The explanation of these and other protective strategies is the objective of this book. We cannot totally avoid the hazards of radiation, not to be sure can we prevent all damage when such exposure occurs, whether this is from medical sources (investigative or therapeutic radiation) or the exposure which can result from such accidents as occurred at Three Mile Island, Chernobyl or Windscale. Nor can it totally stop the effects of the daily exposure to many free radical producing agents in our lives. It can, however, reduce the dangers; slow the damage, and in some cases eliminate the problems associated with some forms of radiation.

Research

One of the chief sources of information about protection from radiation dangers is the research that has gone into space exploration. The Russians have researched the effects, in this regard, of over 25,000 different chemical substances in the search for protection against radiation for their cosmonauts. Professor Izrail Brekhman writes (*Man and Biologically Active Substances*, Pergamon Press, 1980): 'This research resulted in only a small number of substances - radiation protectors - which, on being introduced into animals at a fixed time before irradiation, can to some exstent reduce radiation's injurious effects and increase the animal's survival. Under certain experimental conditions some of the radiation protectors provide 100 per cent survival, whereas control animals die.'

Interestingly, of all the substances found useful in this form of pre-emptive action against known radiation hazards, the herb ginseng was the most effective. This is fine, the professor naturally remarks, if the cosmonaut knows in advance that he is to be exposed to radiation, and can take preventive measures. It is not much use after the event.

However, for those undertaking radiation therapy it is of considerable value, for as we shall see the possibility exists of minimizing dramatically the expected side-effects of this form of treatment. There are other strategies which require implementation if radiation has already occurred, in order to lessen the damage which could take place. All this will be discussed in appropriate sections.

Radiation is everywhere

Over the period of a year people receive radiation from a variety of natural and unnatural sources at a surprising rate. This derives, for example, from cosmic radiation from space. We are protected to a large extent by the atmosphere which filters the rays entering it, but the higher we are in elevation the greater is exposure, and the more time spent outdoors the greater is exposure. Mountain climbers would seem to have a greater average exposure on both counts. Cosmic ray damage is thought to account for as much as 3 per cent of all cancers in man.

How much is a millrem?

As mentioned, the absorbed radiation in man is measured in rems. A typical X-ray would expose the patient to approximately one fiftieth of a rem. This, though, represents the minimum which a quick X-ray view of a bone (for example) may produce. This level does not present great danger to the individual, whereas other forms of X-ray investigation are far more hazardous.

A chest X-ray taken with the machine about two metres away may produce anything from a 50 to 25,000 millirem exposure. The variable will be the skill of the operator, as well as the functioning of the machine. If a series of pictures are taken of the digestive tract where, for example, barium has been swallowed and is being viewed as it passes through the various stages of the digestive process, via fluorscope and X-ray, the rem intake of the body is between 4,000 and 6,000 millirems per minute.

Such a procedure can last for a good twenty minutes, leading to absorption by the individual of as much as 120,000 millirems, which is a great deal when compared to average intakes, from natural sources. A millirem is one thousandth of a rem, so anyone having an X-ray would expect to absorb between 50 millirems and 25,000, for a standard one picture view of a part of the body. Far greater absorption follows other forms of X-ray procedure.

Another example of this is the use of radioactive iodine. This will deliver to the body as much as 10,000 millirems.

How much is too much?

Recent studies, in the USA, on X-ray exposure give the following guidelines as to 'safe' levels of exposure:

Anyone over the age of 18:

No more than 300 millirems (or millirads if you prefer) per week with no more than a total of 5 rems per year (5,000 millirems). Since some of the radiation effects are cumulative, the measurement of lifetime exposure which is acceptable under these guidelines would be ascertained by substracting 18 from the current age, and multiplying by 5. For example, at age 40, the total exposure throughout life should not have exceeded $40 - 18 = 22 \times 5 = 110$ rads, or rems or R of radioactivity.

Anyone under 18:

No more than 100 millirems per year.
(Note rads and rems are not always interchangeable since some forms of radiation such as alpha rays have ten times the biological activity as compared to gamma rays, for example. Thus 1 rad of alpha radiation and 1 rad of gamma radiation, in the same body, would have 10 and 1 rem of effect respectively, on that person).

Absorption of anything between 1 and 100 rems (1,000 to 100,000 millirems) produces the first signs of radiation sickness, which are nausea and vomiting, with usually non-fatal results. A count of 200 R (rad or rem) is enough to produce infertility in both males and females.

We all receive, on average, from natural sources, around 100 millirems of radiation (one tenth of a rem) per year. Airline crews who fly across vast distances are exposed to as much radiation as are nuclear power workers. Such workers, in US nuclear power stations, are advised to receive no more than 3 rems (3,000 millirems) of exposure per three-month period. This translates into no more than 12 rems (12,000 millirems) per year from all sources. This is considerably more than the average individual will be exposed to, unless X-ray procedures such as those mentioned are undertaken, or the occupation involves exposure to other sources.

The symptoms of radiation sickness are fatigue, weakness, loss of appetite, nausea, vomiting, loss of hair, skin changes including altered pigmentation and wrinkling, dilated blood vessels, and gastro-intestinal disturbances in many cases.

Radiation and the unborn child

According to a recent nationwide study in Britain of childhood cancers and background radiation a total (9 months) foetal dose of less than 0.2 rads is more than sufficient to double the risk of an early leukemia death.

The chances of a child having cancer before puberty increases by 50 per cent if the mature foetus receives as little as 1 rem of radiation. This is why X-ray procedures are no longer carried out during pregnancy unless absolutely necessary. If the foetus is exposed to between 2 to 5 rems then the chances of malformation and chromosome damage greatly increase.

Conventional power stations and radiation

Another power station source of radiation derives from conventional plants, rather than the controversial nuclear ones. Heavy metals which are radioactive, such as radon, thorium, radium and polonium are generated in coal burning power stations.

These reach the atmosphere in the fine fly-ash which is discharged from these, and which is not caught, as a rule, by smoke stack filter equipment. Such radioactive heavy metal particles are deposited in the bones of those who breathe them in, where they are likely to remain for the rest of the person's life.

Other sources

Sources of radiation are thought to divide equally between the radiation which is reaching us from space, and from natural materials in soil and rocks, and the man-made sources which are now so widespread. Where we live influences the degree of exposure greatly. This has to do, both with the elevation (how high we are) and also naturally occuring variations in geological factors.

On average we receive about 80 millirems per year from dental and medical sources via diagnostic X-rays. There is a certain residual degree of radiation in the atmosphere, which has been left from nuclear weapon testing in the past. This is thought to add about 5 millirems per year to our total intake. The degree of radiation in the atmosphere, deriving from power plants is thought to add no more than about 1 millirem per year per person, but this is disputed by many who note that emission controls of many power stations are unable to adequately filter radioactive materials in the dust which leaves them.

From other sources, such as luminous watch dials, airport scanners, electron microscopes, building materials such as concrete and granite etc., we may derive a further 4 to 5 millirems per year. Some substances which we consume are unwitting bearers of a radioactive content. Phosphate fertilizers, as used in some commercial orange production, being a source of environment contamination with radioactivity being added to the fruit.

Smoking as a source of radiation

Smoking is also a large contributor to the load or radiation for many people. The amount of radiation detected in cigarette smoke is large. Second-hand smoke, inhaled by people in the same room as the smoker, is equally damaging. A person who smokes 30 cigarettes daily is having the same amount of radiation exposure as someone who has 300 X-rays of their chest each year! The cancer risks associated with the constituents of cigarettes is compounded by the cancer risks which this degree of radiation produces.

The effective doses and thus the potential cancer risks from different types of X-ray examination vary widely. Using the evidence that radiation effects are cumulative (each dose received adding to the harmful effects of all previous doses) the American National Academy of Sciences estimated that a whole-body dose of one rad or rem, received by a million people each year causes between 70 and 500 excess deaths from cancer annually.

Therapeutic radiation

Radiation therapy uses ionizing radiation to damage or destroy tumour cells. It must therefore be appreciated that damage will also occur to normal cells.

The form of the therapeutic radiation varies. It may be in a wave form such as X or gamma rays, or in a corpuscular form, which is composed of electrons or neutrons. Sources could be from natural substances, such as radium, or artificially produced by such means as cobalt-60 or linear acceleration.

High-energy ionizing radiation consists of a very short wave length and this, naturally enough, has great penetration of tissues. Contemporary radiotherapy is carried out with gamma as well as X-rays. X-rays are the electromagnetic ionizing radiation produced by man-made machines, whereas gamma rays may be produced naturally as well as by machines.

In the past only the very low energy beams of kilovoltage X-rays were used. Today very high energy X-rays are provided from megavoltage devices, and these have deep penetration.

The effect of all radiation therapy (and of natural radiation in everyday life) is often to destroy or damage the DNA, the genetic material of the cells being exposed, so that they can no longer reproduce. The effects on the tissues thus treated are instantaneous in some degree (some cells being immediately killed) but effects involving biological change may continue for months, and in some cases where cancer is ultimately produced by such damaged cells, for many years. This is the case also with radiation exposure in general. There will be some short-term effects, but in the main the long-term dangers are the more insidious and worrying.

Varying types of damage

If we examine briefly the short-term, medium-term and long-term damage, instituted by radiotherapy, in different tissues, we will have some idea of the type of injury which radiation is capable of producing. Radiation treatment of the small intestine elicits a response which starts with diarrhoea, colic and malabsorption problems. This is frequently followed by obstruction of the bowel, requiring surgery anything up to ten years later.

Radiation of the stomach initially produces anorexia (loss of appetite), nausea and reduced presence of digestive acids. Ulcers later develop and the end result is frequently chronic gastritis (inflamed stomach).

Colon and rectal radiation leads initially to diarrhoea and colic and is followed by necrosis (death of local tissue) and a slow narrowing and fibrosis of the passage, with lack of flexibility and associated tissue hardness.

Skin irradiation produces initially redness and loss of skin, very much as is noted in severe sunburn. The skin heals with increased pigmentation and tends to discharge or flake later, with the development of ulcers and deep fibrosis, with a general ageing and wasting effect.

These are examples which indicate that the long-term effects, after the initial inflammatory processes have died down, is to harden, age and generally make long-term changes, in structures which affect the function of the organ or region profoundly.

On a lesser scale are the effects of radiation, day by day, from natural and other sources. When such exposure is great, as in accidents at nuclear power plants, then effects similar to those noted in X-ray therapy can be anticipated, but as will be seen when we look further at medical radiation later, there is a good deal of evidence of there being a protective role, against such effects, to be found in specific nutrients.

Among the effects of radiation at the time of its contact with the body are cellular damage, and reduced efficiency of the defence capability of the body. This latter effect is noted in the white blood cells and platelets in the blood, which dramatically decrease in number.

DNA and RNA damage

The effect on the genetic material which instructs cells as to their structure and function, is the one which presents the greatest long-term hazard of ultimately developing a malignancy.

The major American researcher Professor Roger Williams has stated (*Nutrition Against Disease*, Bantam Books, 1980): 'Protein construction (protein synthesis) takes place continuously during our entire lifetime. The structure of proteins is coded in the DNA,s (desoxyribonucleic acid), and the information is carried by messenger RNAs (ribonucleic acids) to the building sites. Possibly as a result of ageing this mechanism may become imperfect. The messenger RNAs may become slightly defective and lead to the production of proteins that are slightly altered – not quite as effective as they should be. The result is that as time goes by the body eventually may reach a point when repair is so imperfect that vital functions are affected.'

Williams continues: 'Mild irritation (with X-rays for example) of animals, causes their lifespan to be decreased in about the same proportion to the amount of radiation used, and that radiation also causes chromosome aberrations. Mutations are in a sense reproductive errors, and the mutagenic effects of X-ray radiation have long been recognized. Since every organism is subject to some radiation this may be regarded as one cause of ageing.'

Repair by the body of radiation damaged DNA is possible, but this will depend on many variables, not least the overall health and nutritional status of the person. Again we will see that we may be able to influence the outcome of the effects of radiation, beneficially, by nutritional methods.

Short and long term changes

The effects of all forms of excessive radiation especially those derived from exposure to nuclear devices or accidents are operative over a long period. In any large group of people, so affected, the following sequence could be anticipated:

The first notable effect occurs within a few days of exposure to massive radiation, sometimes within hours.

The central nervous system of those massively overdosed is destroyed and death occurs.

Those with lower doses are likely to escape initial death but may die after several weeks as gastro-intestinal damage produces its effects.

If a lower doseage was experienced the individuals may not experience gastro-intestinal damage, but the bone marrow may be so damaged as to produce death a month or so after exposure.

Those that survive these initial severe effects may suffer diseases such as leukemia, especially in children, a few years after exposure. Deaths from such causes continue for about ten years before peaking and reducing in numbers of those exposed.

Some ten years after exposure there will be a rise in the incidence of cancers amongst the survivors. Such forms as breast, thryroid, lung, stomach, liver, large intestine, bone, oesophagus, small intestine, bladder, pancreas, rectum and lymphatic tissues will develop. In frequency they will fall roughly in the order described. Finally the genetic damage caused by radiation remains. Death, disability and malformation will be the legacy for many of the unborn children of the people exposed to such massive radiation exposure as took place at Chernobyl.

Let us examine the degree of radiation exposure required to produce these extreme degrees of damage. Between 0 and

100 rems produces nausea and vomiting. This degree of exposure is seldom fatal.

Remember that the most recent descriptions of radiation strength, as it affects the body, speak of sieverts rather than rems. 100 rems equals one sievert.

Between 100 and 200 rems produces slightly depressed white cell count and is seldom fatal in the short-term, but increases the likelihood of cancer later.

Between 200 and 600 rems exposure causes a severe depression of white blood cells within four to six weeks. The skin will be blotched and there is a fifty per cent chance of death resulting.

Between 600 and 1,000 rems exposure produces even more marked depression of white blood cells, blotched skin and severe gastro-intestinal symptoms within four to six weeks. There is a greater than 80 per cent chance of death resulting.

Between 1,000 and 5,000 rems of exposure produces diarrhoea, fever, blood changes of a dramatic nature and, within a week or two, a virtual 100 per cent certainty of death.

Everyday radiation effects

Whilst the results described above relate to severe exposure to radiation, we should be aware of the daily toll resulting from mild radiation effects. We will look at the damage exerted by free radical agents in the next chapter. These can cause local tissue damage anywhere in the body. One effect of this is to produce what is called cross-linkage. When normal tissue structures link with others in an abnormal manner, they lose flexibility and suppleness and appear to age. Indeed this is the normal ageing process, speeded up by free radical damage. Apart from the small amount of naturally occurring damage of this sort the external contact of the body with radiation is a major element in the process.

When we are young this can to an extent be reversed by enzyme activity. As we age the process appears to be going on more quickly than the repair measures can cope with.

Nutritional support is a major method of improving this

state of affairs and slowing down the ageing process. The nutrients needed are largely those which protect against free radical damage, and therefore from radiation damage. These are numerous, and many of them are anti-oxidants, such as vitamins A, C and E, as well as amino acids, and the minerals zinc and selenium.

Prevention of damage?

Not all of the harmful effects of radiation are preventable, but some can be prevented and others minimized, by the methods which we will outline later, especially those effects which follow the lower levels of exposure.

Gastro-intestinal damage may be helped and limited by the use of substances which lock onto the radioactive materials in the bowel. This is a major strategy which will be described. The other effect of radiation which is amenable to some degree of control is that which occurs as a result of free radical damage, triggered by the radiation. This is the second nutritional strategy which will be discussed and outlined.

We have, in these two approaches, something concrete which can be done and which can be shown, by experimental evidence, to be effective to a very large degree, depending upon how much tissue damage has already occurred at the time of commencing such positive action.

There is also the strategy which may be adopted by anyone who has advance knowledge of the likelihood of exposure to radiation. Anyone having diagnostic X-ray procedures done, or who is receiving medical treatment involving radiation, or who is working in an environment which leads to excessive exposure, can take such preventative action. This also will be discussed in a later section.

Irradiation of food

A modern method of food preservation, which is officially described as safe, is irradiation. Is this harmful to us? There is little evidence of such food when eaten being able to harm the body as a result of it being radioactive in any sense. However, as we have noted one of the main anti-oxidants which protect the body against radiation, and free radical damage, is vitamin

E. Indeed this is a major part played by vitamin E in the economy of the body as we will see.

When food is irradiated, to give it a long shelf-life, there is an overall vitamin loss of between 20 and 80 per cent. However, vitamin E is totally destroyed, and it has been found that when such food has vitamin E added to it, after irradiation, in an attempt to restore natural levels, it is again destroyed by contact with the irradiated food. This is hardly a confidence boosting thought as far as the nutritive values of such foods are concerned. Such foods are a major source of free radicals.

Incidentally, other processing methods such as freezing, cooking or simply leaving foods open to the air, all destroy vitamin E. Since this is the most potent anti-oxidant available we should ensure adequate intake as part of a defensive strategy.

There is something to be said for attempting to monitor the environment in which we live, for actually checking on local radiation levels in the home, work place and in the food and drink being consumed. Guidance will be given as to how this might be achieved.

Radiation is not going to go away. It has been with man from the dawn of time. Unfortunately levels will continue to rise, for a variety of reasons, some obvious others less so. The atmosphere itself is now damaged by man-made factors, so that its efficiency as a filter of cosmic rays is declining. Already scientists are discussing the new hazards to man of the disappearance of part of the ozone layer over the poles. This is a shield against some forms of radiation which will increase as a result of the reduced shield. One of the reasons for this loss is the emission of supersonic aircraft. Another is thought to relate to the propellants in aerosol sprays. Whatever the reasons, this shield is vital to normal life on earth, and must be protected if we are to avoid having to live in a vastly different manner, with considerably increased radiation reaching us when outdoors. Man-made radiation will continue, inevitably, and we must take what precautions we can.

In the final chapter of the book will be found some aspects of non-ionizing radiation, the health effects of which we are as yet not clear about. The risks of radiation from ionized particles are, however, much more clearly established.

When an exposure is described as a whole body exposure, this indicates that it is assumed that each part of the body has received that degree of exposure (say one rem). This is far more serious than one rem exposure to just a part of the body.

In assessing means of protection we are concerned with ionizing radiation. This is the form of radiation which occurs when tiny charged particles tear themselves away from the nucleus of the atom of a substance, and leave that atom with a positive electrical charge. This makes it an ion, and is the characteristic of high energy radiation.

In the following chapter we will look at what happens when ionic forms of energy transform elements of normal physiology into free radical oxidants, which have a powerful potential for harm, and we will investigate means by which this damage can be controlled.

2. Free Radicals – The Consequences Of Radiation

So that we can see just what anti-radiation benefits are available from nutritional sources we must look at the ways in which radiation causes damage within our bodies, and the major tissue effect which has to be considered is that caused by free radical oxidation.

In order to understand the nature and effects in the body of free radicals (more accurately called free oxidizing radicals or FORs) we have to look at aspects of life which at first do not appear to be connected with radiation.

FORs and oxygen

We are bathed from the cradle to the grave in oxygen. Without it, for only a few minutes, life becomes impossible for us, yet its very qualities carry the potential for damage. Oxygen reacts in a variety of ways with other molecules. Consider the effect of bleach on the hair or skin of a person, or on material. Bleach is hydrogen peroxide, and it may come as a surprise to know that our own white blood cells produce hydrogen peroxide almost constantly in their defence of our bodies against invading micro-organisms.

Hydrogen peroxide is a free oxidizing radical, and so that this effective defence measure causes no damage to the body cells themselves there is an efficient de-activating procedure which neutralizes the FORs and which takes place within a split second of their activation.

The life of a free radical is, ideally, very short indeed under healthy conditions. If, however, free radical production is very high, or if the de-activating process is impaired or unable to cope with the sheer number of FORs present, then tissue damage will result.

FORs: where do they come from?

Pesticides, smog, exhaust fumes etc. in the atmosphere are all potent sources of FORs. Consider the effect on the eyes when in an area where there is high atmospheric pollution. They smart and, within a short time, become watery and irritated. This is the effect on the eye surface of free radical activity. The tears carry the antioxidants and this relieves the stinging and smarting effects. Similar changes occur when the free radicals in polluted air are inhaled. The mucous membranes of the nose and throat are affected, causing the nose to run and the sinuses to become inflamed, and coughing of protective mucus from the lungs will start. This is all in response to free radical activity that is threatening the biological structures with which it is in contact.

The smell of newly painted surfaces, the fumes from dry cleaning processes, a host of chemicals in everyday use in the home, office and industry; all are highly charged with free radical oxidizers, and the effect of solar energy on all of these chemicals is to increase oxidizing activity since it ionizes them.

And what of food?

A lot of foods are potential carriers or producers of free radical activity. All oils and fats, when they become rancid or altered by heat, produce free radical oxidation. A variety of drinks and foods contain substances called methylxanthines. Caffeine is one of these. When a methylxanthine is consumed it produces the body a breakdown product called xanthine, and this in turn produces a chemical free radical called a superoxide.

Of course, there is also tobacco smoke. As mentioned in the previous chapter, cigarette smoke is radioactive through its heavy metal polonium content. Also in tobacco smoke are carbon monoxide and nitrogen oxide (both found in smog) which abnormally oxidize body fats through the production of free radicals; turning them into potential cancer inducing agents.

There are defence mechanisms in the body which can deactivate superoxides, but these are sometimes simply overwhelmed, either by a surplus of superoxides with which to deal, or because of inadequate numbers of superoxide quenchers (also called free radical scavengers), or a combination of both. Nutritious food is the body's primary source of the materials with which it fights such enemies.

Two of the defending substances in the body which deal with such superoxides are enzymes called superoxide dismutase (SOD) and glutathione peroxidase.

Different types of FORs

Among the different chemicals which fall under the description of free oxidizing radicals are ozone (O_3), superoxide (O_2), hydrogen peroxide (H_2O_2), hypochlorite (OC1), hydroxyl (OH), and organic peroxides (ROOH). All of these have the ability to donate an electron when a chemical reaction is taking place. Superoxide (O_2) plus water (H_2O) equals hydrogen peroxide ($2H_20_2$) plus e^-. It is the extra electron (e^-) which is a further potential for harm in the body. These can split the strong double bonds which link normally stable materials in the body.

Ageing as a consequence

The double helix which forms DNA, the genetic coding material of every cell of the body, is held together by a double sulphur bond. There are other double bonds which make this a stable structure, but these bonds can be broken by oxidation.

Once DNA is damaged in this way it will no longer be able to provide the cell with accurate information. This impairs the function of the cell and harms its ability to synthesize protein. It is no longer able to reproduce precisely, as when unharmed, and subsequent cells produced by damaged DNA instruction, and impaired protein synthesis, will be abnormal.

Such changes, which occur in all life forms as part of the normal ageing process, are speeded up dramatically by free radical activity. Ageing and the process of cross-linking of tissues is a major result of free radical damage to cells. These changes, as well as the interference with protein synthesis which is part of the free radical damage, and the alteration of DNA, represents the areas of damage which nutritional methods can influence beneficially and, in many cases, prevent.

More serious consequences

If an acceleration of ageing were not enough, then the other potential danger from DNA damage is of profound significance. Once the genetic coding is altered, the cells which reproduce thereafter may well be malignant. Mutant cells triggering the processes of cancer are the potential results of free radical oxidation of normal cells.

The changes which occur in the arteries, and which end up as atherosclerosis and cardiovascular disease, are also often the result of FOR activity. Blood which carries a high level of what is called low density lipoprotein (LDL) – which is a carrier of cholesterol – has a high potential for such damage. This is thought to result from impurities in the cholesterol which produces FOR activity. A diet rich in saturated fats and sugars is likely to produce such high levels of LDLs.

High energy radiation damages and kills by generating free radicals in living organisms. Hydroxyl radicals are the most potent oxidants known and are capable of attacking any of the body cells. These are largely produced by radiation.

First described in the 1950's by Dr Denham Harman, the activity of free radicals in the body results in what he calls 'internal radiation'. 'Spontaneous mutations, cancer and ageing can be looked on as a result of continuous "internal radiation".' There is, however, a bright side to all this. There are protective factors which are readily available.

Protection factors

One of the major discoveries in recent years concerning nutritional protection against both cancer and heart disease relates to the trace element selenium. Selenium is a major antioxidant and is a component of the free radical de-activator gluthathione peroxidase. This is one of the substances which we will return to later, as it is a vital part of an anti-radiation damage programme.

Further FOR activity results

Allergies, and self-allergies (the so-called auto-immune diseases, such as rheumatoid arthritis) are also thought to involve the activites of FORs in the body cells. The resulting inflammatory processes are thought to take place in such conditions where an antigen (something to which the body is sensitive) combines with a normal cell wall in a process in which FORs take part. Leslie Kenton, in her book *Ageless Ageing*, (Century Arrow, 1986), states: 'Much of the damage from radiation comes because of radioactivity's ability to steal electrons from water molecules in the body, turning them into hydroxyl radicals which in turn get together to form peroxides. These peroxides emasculate anti-oxidant enzymes such as catalase by damaging their sulphydral groups. When sufficient sulphur amino acids are present in the body then sufficient sulphydral groups are available to be sacrificed by combining with free radicals and peroxides, so that antioxidant enzymes remain protected to carry out their jobs.'

This is a clue to further protection for the body from the damage of radiation and free radicals. The ample presence in the body of sulphur-rich amino acids such as methionine and cysteine, and the amino acid-selenium compound glutathione, provide just such protection, and these will be returned to in a later section. Let us not lose sight of the fact that it is free radical activity which damages and destroys the DNA, and the protein synthesizing ability of cells. It thus produces cross-linkages in tissues which make them older and tougher than they should be.

Much of the damaging effect of radiation is the direct result of free radical activity. Fortunately there has been a vast amount of research into methods of providing the body with antioxidant nutrients which protect against this.

Part of the free radical activity is the result of excess metal in the body: lead, copper, cadmium, aluminium, for instance, are all capable of oxidation to some extent and to the production of free radicals. Cigarette smoke is a potent producer of free radicals in the body, and this goes for both the smoker and those obliged to inhale second-hand smoke due to unavoidable proximity with smokers. Alcohol is another source of these destructive elements. Indeed, all toxic substances, to some extent, involve free radical activity and damage.

A defence against such damaging free-radical activity in the body should therefore consist of a reduction or elimination of cigarettes, alcohol and exposure to toxic substances. Added to this there should be an increase in the intake of antioxidants which protect against free radical effects.

As Pearson and Shaw (*Life Extension*, Warner Books, 1981) say: 'It is possible to prevent much of this damage by taking supplements of nutrients which provide protection against free radicals. Many of these nutrients have even extended the life-span of experimental animals. These anti-free-radical nutrients (also called antioxidants) include Vitamins A, C, E, B_1, B_5, B_6; the amino acid cysteine (found in eggs and sometimes in health food stores) the triamino acid-cysteine containing compound, glutathione; phenolic and atecholic amino acids like tyrosine and L-Dopa; catechols as found in bananas and potatoes; phenolics found in grapes and other fruits; the minerals zinc and selenium; bioflavonoids, and synthetic antioxidants.'

There are also other nutrient protection aids to the potential damage of radiation itself, and these include extracts from seaweed, such as algin, and the common constituent of fruits and vegetables (apples especially) pectin. As mentioned, there is also protection to be derived from sources such as the herb ginseng, much used in Russia for this purpose. A further strategy in protecting against radiation damage is to enhance the cell wall structures which are the initial area of damage cuased by the free radicals.

It makes sense to not only minimize exposure to factors which cause the free radicals, and to include nutrients which de-activate these (antioxidants) and to eat safe substances which will speed the transit of radioactive material through the body (special fibres such as pectin) but also to strengthen those structures which are most vulnerable.

This latter defence is achieved by the use of a number of nutrients, including essential fatty acids which are vital in the construction of the cell membranes and the intercellular cement. Altogether, apart from avoiding the obvious hazards presented by both radiation in general and free radicals in particular, the use of selected nutrients can be a major contributory element in defence against radiation's potential for damaging the body.

This is the case in general exposure from atmospheric and environmental contamination as well as in specific instances such as radiation applied diagnostically or therapeutically in medicine.

This approach is the major part of the strategy outlined in this book, and I will examine individually the most important of the defensive antioxidant and anti-free radical nutrients in order to establish the options open to those who would wish to apply such measures to themselves and their families. Radiation kills through free radical activity (largely). We must defend against this.

Such a programme should include the *avoidance* of cigarette smoke and other smoke; contact with petrocarbons and the vapours of these; alcohol; excessive fats whether these be saturated or polyunsatured; contact in air or food with heavy metals (lead, mercury, cadmium etc.). And there should be *increased intake* of antioxidant nutrients such as Vitamin A, C, E, B_5 and B_6, selenium, zinc, amino acids such as cysteine, histidine, taurine etc., those most useful herbs ginseng and garlic, pectins and algins etc. which bind and speed the elimination of radioactive materials in the bowel, and those nutrients which are known to help in the construction of more efficient cell membranes, such as essential fatty acids.

Above all, we should be aware of the substances in our environment which pose threats to life and health and, without becoming obsessed, we should avoid these.

Nutritional support should involve both eating the most desirable foods, as well as the judicious use of supplements which are readily available from health food stores and pharmacies. These should be used regularly by anyone in contact with undesirable sources of free radical activity, whether this be through radiation or any of the other sources of free radical activity. Eating foods which are whole and fresh, and as free as possible from chemical contamination (pesticides etc.), is also suggested.

3. PROTECTING AGAINST EFFECTS OF RADIOTHERAPY

Although in this chapter I concentrate on aspects of radiotherapy, the conclusions which are drawn are of value in all cases of radiation damage. It it can be shown that a particular nutrient can reduce potential for damage from X-ray therapy, then this is of vital importance to anyone exposed to other sources of radiation.

The medical treatment of cancers of many sorts involves the use of radiotherapy. There is, though, debate as to the long-term desirability of this in some forms of cancer, such as breast cancer, where long-term survival rates appear to be no better and, in some studies, are actually worse where radiation has been used.

In a speech delivered to the National Cancer Conference in 1968 Dr Philip Ruben, then chief of radiotherapy at the University of Rochester Medical School, stated that the clinical evidence and statistical data, derived from the study of numerous reviews of this procedure, proved that no increase in survival rates had been achieved by the use of radiotherapy. Dr Vera Peters of Princess Margaret Hospital, Toronto, informed the same Conference that, despite the much publicized improvements in radiotherapy and surgery techniques, there had been no true improvement in the mortality figures for breast cancer sufferers over the previous thirty years.

This is apparently contradicted by trials in England in which, over a ten year period, women receiving X-ray therapy for breast cancer, had fewer recurrences than those who had no such treatment. However, different research using other criteria, whilst confirming fewer reappearances in breast cancer in the treated women, showed that over a period of ten years, more of these women died of other causes. Swiss experts are known to believe that stopping routine radiotherapy in cases of breast cancer would actually increase survival rates. The debate continues and is unlikely to be easily resolved, since those receiving the therapy are not a standardized product. They differ in many ways from one another, and not least of the differences is nutritional.

Brenda Kidman points out in *A Gentle Way with Cancer* (Century, 1983): 'Small doses of X-ray given at intervals over a long period eventually add up to the same as one large dose, and it is difficult to predict what the delayed side-effects of this might be.' This element, of radiation being cumulative in its potential for damage, is well worth re-emphasizing. Each exposure is added to all previous exposures. True some of the damage may have been repaired in the interim, but radioactive material which has entered the body and become locked into the bone or other tissues (thyroid for example) is added to by each subsequent exposure to more radiation. Refer to the outline of radiation damage given in Chapter 1 which describes both the short and the long term hazards and likely sequence of symptoms.

In some cases there is obvious benefit derived from radiotherapy, but the overall statistics imply that there is no standard reaction to such methods, with much depending upon the stage of the disease as well as on many intangibles, such as the nutritional and mental state of the patient. This degree of variability in response to therapy has been shown by distinguished scientists to be capable of being altered quite easily. A number of these have shown that by simple manipulation of the diet it is possible to change dramatically the manner in which the body responds to radiotherapy. Thus without becoming involved in the debate in the overall desirability, or otherwise, of radiotherapy, it is the intention in this chapter to stress the ways in which (a) radiotherapy may be received with the minimum of danger and damage to the individual receiving it, and (b) radiotherapy may be more likely to be beneficial in its antitumour effects.

It is well established that radiation destroys (partly by free radical activity) a major number of vitamins in the body, including the antioxidant vitamins A, C, E as well as K, a number of the B vitamins and also essential fatty acids (sometimes called vitamin F). Let us examine some of the ways in which it has been shown that nutrient supplementation and manipulation of the diet, has been able to improve the health of people undergoing radiotherapy.

In March 1972 (*Journal of the National Cancer Institute,* Washington) animal studies showed that if vitamin A was injected at the same time as radiotherapy was performed, it was possible to increase the radiation dose by around 20 per cent without any increase in local tissue damage. The scientists stated that if it were shown to be possible to safely increase radiation exposure in human patients, the results in terms of tumour destruction would be greatly enhanced.

This trial is an echo of human experience noted some ten years earlier in which over fifty women, who were undergoing radiation therapy for cancer of the cervix, were placed on a diet high in vitamin A for a week prior to therapy. When assessed three weeks after treatment, those women who had been on the special diet before therapy showed a favourable response of 97 per cent or more. Those women not having the vitamin-rich diet were found to have the expected rate of improvement of just over 60 per cent. Vitamin A, an antioxidant which protects the vital mucous membranes of the body, is seen to have a potential for minimizing the damage to general healthy tissue as well as enhancing the anti-tumour effect of radiotherapy.

Emanuel Cheraskin's work

Professor Emeritus, Emanuel Cheraskin, of the University of Alabama, has studied many aspects of nutrition in relation to health. Together with colleagues he studied the effect of diet upon the radiation response of patients with cancer of the uterus. He explains the desired effects of radiation: 'The impact of ionizing radiation on cancer may be conveniently considered in two categories (1) the direct effect on tumour cells, and (2) the indirect effect on the tumour, mediated through alterations in the host and the tumour bed.'

The success of radiotherapy is measured by the product of both of these body changes. When deciding whether or not radiotherapy is successful both the characteristics of the tumour itself, as well as the characteristics of the person who has the tumour are considered, in order to note results thus far, and to predict the likely outcome of therapy.

Cheraskin and co-workers examined the radiation response in a random group of patients with cervical cancer, and also in a group of women of similar age who had been placed on a relatively high protein, low refined carbohydrate, diet with multivitamin and mineral supplementation. The two groups were then compared as to their overall response to radiation.

The diet which the patients who were receiving supplements were placed on consisted of the following: (*Note:* this began one week before radiation therapy and continued until three weeks after its termination):

Animal protein such as fish, meat, fowl, or eggs was encouraged at each meal. Carbohydrates of low nutritional value such as snacks, desserts, white flour and all sugar, were virtually eliminated. The researchers point out that this was done for a variety of reasons not least because it provided optimal intake of vitamins, minerals and protein. In addition multivitamin-multimineral capsules were given which provided nutrients in excess of normally accepted levels of requirement.

Whilst this group was following the diet and having radiotherapy a similar number of women were having treatment of the same kind but these received no dietary advice or supplements.

The results were of great significance. The group which received no advice dietetically had a positive radiation response of 63.3 per cent. This is regarded as poor since the standard point at which results are though of as 'good', is when there is a 70 per cent response. This 63.3 per cent result represented the average result of the group of nearly thirty women. In arriving at this average it should be noted that nearly half the women in this group failed to achieve a 70 per cent response rate.

Of the nearly thirty women receiving radiotherapy, and also following the dietary advice, the average good response was 97.5 per cent. This group had no poor responders and the average mentioned was derived from a lowest response of 91 per cent to highest of 100 per cent. This latter result being achieved in many of these patients. Every subject in the experimental group (those getting vitamins etc) demonstrated a favourable score using standard medical criteria for analysing the response.

The researchers commented on the fact that amongst those who received no advice at all, whilst the average was poor, and over half had very poor responses, there were some good responders, and that this probably relates to their own nutritional habit. These were not analysed since this group was left on their own in this area.

The complete vindication of an improved diet of this type offering dramatic differences in response to radiation deserves wide recognition. Unfortunately little follow up work has been done on this research which indicates methods which could well be copied in every radiotherapy department in the world, with very little effort and to great advantage.

There has been other confirmation of this type of research. For example, in Houston in 1975, Dr Edward Copeland proved that hyperalimentation (optimum feeding) was successful in replenishing the strength of cancer patients who were having radiotherapy and chemotherapy.

Dr Cheraskin's research showed that just a week on an optimum diet was enough to boost the response of a patient receiving radiotherapy and that this led to every patient in the trial responding well (over 90 per cent of the cancer cells destroyed by radiation treatment on average and many achieving 100 per cent cell destruction). Dr Copeland's research showed the same thing, and even when patients could not respond adequately, the better nutrition enabled them to be more comfortable in the last days of their lives. Adelle Davis, the American nutritionist and author states that: 'Many harmful substances are formed in the body by the destruction of malignant tissue (by X-ray or chemotherapy) and that the liver will more readily do its work of detoxification if vitamin C and vitamin E are generously supplied. This helps prevent skin burning, pain and scarring.'

Recall that vitamin C and E are antioxidants and reduce free radical activity. This is part of the protective support which their ample presence ensures.

Dr Robert Klenner states in *A Physician's Handbook of Orthomolecular Medicine* (Keats, 1977): 'Massive employment of vitamin C will make possible prolonged radiation therapy in many cases. It will also prevent radiation burns.' This is of considerable importance to all those receiving radiation, since burns are a major side-effect, with often painful and disfiguring consequences. Methods of safe supplementation of 'massive' doses of vitamin C will be outlined in a later section.

When we are stressed or ill the requirements for certain nutrients rises dramatically. Professor Dickerson of the University of Sussex Nutrition Unit, has shown radiation therapy raises the body's need for vitamin C and B complex by 300 per cent. The work of Professor Roger Williams (Biochemical Individuality) has shown that we all have an individual need for all nutrients which differs between people – markedly in some cases. In order to maintain normal functions in the body, the difference in requirement in any group of ten or fifteen people, for a particular nutrient may differ by as much as 700 per cent. This means that the requirement of the person in the group with the lowest need for, say vitamin C (as demonstrated by chiochemical analysis of tissues and fluids in the body) will be seven times less than the requirement of the person in the group with the highest need. These variations in need are genetically acquired, as well as relating to current health, stress and other factors.

Thus, when Professor Dickerson states that radiation produces a threefold increase in requirement for B complex vitamins and vitamin C, we should realize that this would be a variable amount depending upon the individual needs of that person at the outset. Fortunately there are simple methods for achieving optimum amounts of such nutrients as vitamin C and these will be discussed along with the best method for 'saturating' the tissues with this vital antioxidant, later in the book.

Dealing with nausea

One of the earliest symptoms noted by anyone with radiation sickness is nausea. It is standard medical practice to provide vitamin B_6 to anyone with such symptoms after radiation therapy. Many radiologists now provide it before treatment as a preventive measure, which seems a more sensible approach rather than waiting for the symptoms and then acting. In the amounts required, vitamin B_6 (pyridoxine) is completely safe (it also often controls the nausea of morning sickness during pregnancy). Although not an antioxidant itself the body converts a common amino acid methionine into the powerful antioxidant cystathione, with the help of vitamin B_6. If the diet contains excessive amounts of methionine (say from a rich diet of meat) and inadequate B_6, which is commonly the case, then instead of being able to manufacture the helpful and protective antioxidant out of the methionine, the body ends up with increased levels of oxidizing materials which are thought to take part in the process which leads to atherosclerosis.

Among the many reasons for B_6 deficiency is that it is destroyed by alcohol, cigarettes and the contraceptive pill, as well as by excessive cooking. Thus we should realize that simply having an adequate intake of antioxidants is not enough. Other complementary nutrients must accompany them.

The two ways which X-rays damage cells are the direct effect on the DNA genetic coding material and the initiation of free radical activity which disrupts cell membrane structures, interferes with protein synthesis, initiates cross-linkage of tissues and accelerates the ageing process.

Vitamin E protects the lysosome membrances of the cells and thus is a highly valuable part of an anti-radiation damage programme for anyone receiving radiotherapy, but we will consider individual nutrients in a later section and provide details of their other roles, as well as the best sources.

Other research evidence comes from the USA where Florida-based Dr Boris Sokaloff reduced the death rate in animals receiving radiation from X-rays from 80 per cent to 10 per cent, by giving them bioflavonoids (so-called vitamin P). It is known that these substances protect the capillaries and the fine intercellular material of the body, and this may be the role it plays in reducing the harmful effects of radiation.

Similar animal trials in Hungary show that calcium pantothenate (vitamin B_5) is capable of acting in a protective capacity. X-rays produced only half the damage in those treated with B_5 when it was given before exposure. German studies in the mid- 1970s involved an attempt to protect women against the effects of radiation therapy. The women in question were being treated for inoperable cancer with a combination of radium and cobalt 60. Some were given no nutrient supplements whereas others received 20g of pollen, three times daily. A variety of beneficial effects were noted in the women receiving this, including improvement in many aspects of their blood state. Patients on pollen had half as much nausea, and almost no lack of appetite, fewer sleep disorders, reduced inflammation, and their overall condition worsened at a third of a rate of those not receiving pollen. No conclusions were reaced as to what it was in pollen which offered these benefits and protection, but the results are proof of the possibility of improving the status of patients at almost any stage of their illness even when radiotherapy is being used, by dietary measures. The research outlined above is clear indication that radiation damage may be minimized, and radiation effects enchanced, in an anti-tumour role by nutrition.

These conclusions should be borne in mind as we move on to develop the overall anti-radiation-damage strategy, using nutritional methods, in subsequent chapters.

General nutritional advice

The general advice below, as to dosages, etc. is a guide which should be understood to be non-specific since doses must remain a matter of individual needs. In general anyone receiving radiation therapy should ensure that overall nutrition is good, with adequate protein and minimal refined carbohydrate (white flour products and sugar of all sorts).

A strong formula vitamin B complex tablet should be taken

daily before radiotherapy (which should contain no less than 50mg each of vitamins B_5 and B_6 – pantothenic acid, which may be described as calcium pantothenate, and pyridoxine).

At least 3g daily of vitamin C should be taken in divided doses and more if possible (see Chapter 5 for details on reaching tissue saturation of vitamin C).

In addition the intake of bioflavonoids should be ensured. Some forms of vitamin C are formulated with bioflavonoids. If this is the case, then taking one ensures the taking of the other. If not, then additional bioflavonoids are required separately (in plants vitamin C usually occurs together with bioflavonoids).

In most good formulations of this sort there would be approximately 20 times as much vitamin C in a tablet as bioflavonoids. In dealing with radiation problems, however, where it is desirable to provide excessive but safe amounts of both these vital nutrients, a formulation should be used in which the ratio is only about 3 or 2½ to 1 (vitamin C to bioflavonoid). Such a formula is available from Lamberts, PO Box 1, Tunbridge wells, Kent, as 'Ultra Vitamin C 500mg Complex'. This contains half a gram of vitamin C and 100mg of lemon bioflavonoids, 30mg of hesperidin complex, and 50mg of rutin (another form of bioflavonoid).

Also, 100 iu of vitamin E (not in cases of breast cancer) and 25,000 iu of vitamin A should be taken daily. A good formula multimineral tablet should be obtained, which ensures that daily intake exceeds the recommended daily allowance (RDA) of the minerals mentioned, by at least 100 per cent. (Note the RDA is the amount suggested as a minimum by health authorites.)

Calcium and magnesium should be taken (perhaps for economy in the form of bone meal tablets or dolomite tablets) so that not less than one gram of calcium, and half a gram of magnesium, are consumed daily. Also, 100 mcg of selenium should be taken daily. Pollen tablets made in Sweden with the brand name 'Cernilton', should be taken in appropriate doses (Note: in the trial discussed above, up to 60g daily was utilized. This is unnecessary if other nutrients are being used which support the protective function of the substances in pollen. The dosage recommended on the container should be followed or exceeded by doubling it, no more, if other nutritional supplements are being taken as advised.)

Finally essential fatty acids should be obtained from a source such as linseed oil or evening primrose oil (Efamol) capsules, at a dosage of 1,000mg daily.

All the above should be taken with food. Additional anti-radiation protection can be achieved by using the amino-acids, cysteine, glutathione etc. as described later in this book.

Ideally the nutrient programme should be begun at least one week prior to radiotherapy and continued for the duration of the therapy at the very least. The only likely side-effect is that diarrhoea may result from excessive use of vitamin C. This is discussed on page 65. Once treatment is over, continuation is still desirable, but at a substantially reduced dosage, such as that outlined as a General Maintenance Protection Programme in Chapter 6.

4. Nutritional Removal Of Radioactive Material From The Body

It makes sense to attempt to remove as much in the way of radioactive material which may have entered the body, before it can do any more damage than it already has done. This should not of course preclude co-ordinated and simultaneous attempts to minimize such damage, by nutritional methods, which address the dangers associated with free radical activity, DNA damage, cell membrane damage, protein synthesis problems, etc. as mentioned in the previous chapter.

There are a number of favoured sites in which radioactive material may lodge. Bone is one such site, as is the thyroid, for radioactive iodine. The digestive tract is another area through which radioactive material is likely to travel. These sites should receive attention in any attempt to dislodge unwelcome radioactive material which might be present, as a result of ingestion of contaminated food or drink, or of absorption through penetration of the body, or through inhalation.

Strontium 90 and Iodine 131 as well as Cesium 137 are the

likeliest forms of radioactive contamination to enter the body as a result of nuclear accidents. It should be remembered that Strontium 90 and Cesium 137 are likely to find their way into the top-soil of an area thus affected, and that it will take decades for the substances to decay to safe levels. Iodine 131 has a shorter life, but once an area has been contaminated the prevention programmes which are outlined in this book are desirable for years, in order to minimize the risks.

Any radioactive material absorbed into the body, via food or through inhalation, circulates through the blood stream. Some of this is likely to become bound to bone and other tissues, as well as continually recirculating and passing through the gastro-intestinal tract. This presents the best opportunity for physically removing the radioactive material.

Algin from seaweed

Substances such as sodium alginate contain the fibre algin, which is derived from seaweed. This is quite indigestible but has an affinity for Strontium 90, which it binds itself to as the algin passes through the digestive tract. This is then excreted during bowel movements. Research into its efficacy in animals exposed to radiation was conducted in Canada at McGill University, Montreal, under the sponsorship of the Atomic Energy Commission. This research showed that algin, in sufficiently high dosages, offers protection from Strontium 90 of between 50 and 80 per cent. For obvious reasons it was not possible to test the efficacy in humans, but there is no reason whatever to suppose that the behaviour of algin would be any different in humans than it is in animals, since it is indigestible in both (i.e. it passes through the bowel without being absorbed at all) and since Strontium 90 circulates through the gastro-intestinal tract in both man and animals once it is absorbed into the body.

Algin is available in the form of sodium alginate from some UK suppliers (see page 87) in powder form or in half gram doses. Since the requirement, in order to effectively produce the same results as in the animals in the trials, would be around 10g daily this would entail the taking of some 20 tablets, of this type daily. In a situation in which exposure to

Strontium 90 was known to have taken place this should be done, or the equivalent amount taken in powder form (see below).

Kelp

Another source of algin is kelp which is found in powder and tablet form in most health food stores. The amount of algin in such tablets is not always stated, however, and fairly high doses may be required to achieve good results. This is discussed below, as is the presence in kelp of the element iodine.

The eating of seaweed, such as the dried Japanese seaweeds kombu, nori, hijiki, arame or wakame (among others) which are available from many wholefood and specialists shops, also offers a fine source of algin. If sodium alginate is available in power form then the amount required would be contained in approximately two tablespoonfuls daily. According to Mark Bricklin (*Natural Healing*, Rodale Press, 1976) algin should be taken up to four times a daily since it is desirable for there to always be some in the intestinal tract to do its job of binding radioactive material. He says: 'Algin must be mixed with sufficient fluid to get it down. Some kind of thick soup is best. If you are using tablets, which usually weigh only half a gram, chew up six or eight, and swallow with milk four times daily.' This would certainly provide an ample intake of algin, if a rather excessive amount of milk. Since algin remains undigested by the body, it has no toxic limit.

A form of algin which is recommended is that combined with selenium, as selenium alginate (available from Larkhall Laboratories, see page 87 for details of address). There could, however, be selenium toxicity if very high doses were taken for very long, and so selenium alginate intake should not exceed four tablets per day for longer than a week or so. Other sources of algin should be sought as an addition to this formula which combines 50mg of selenium with 500mg of alginate, together with additional vitamin B_6, vitamin E, magnesium and lecithin; all of which are highly useful in anti-radiation and detoxification terms.

Iodine

Another advantage of the use of seaweed, either eaten as a food or taken in the form of powder or as kelp tablets, is that it provides a good source of iodine for the body. This protects the thyroid gland against uptake of Iodine 131, the radioactive form, which is so damaging to thyroid function and which threatens life itself. Since kelp provides the opportunity for reducing Strontium 90 absorption through the bowel, as well as reducing Iodine 131 uptake by the thyroid, it is a highly desirable addition to the programme of prevention of radiation damage.

Powdered kelp can be added to soups or savoury drinks or can be swallowed with water, or taken as tablets. It is available from Larkhall Laboratories in powdered form. A satisfactorally high dosage would be derived by the taking of two tablespoons of kelp powder or granules daily, or the taking of ten tablets daily (ideally deep sea or Pacific kelp). Such a dosage would only be necessary in the case of actual exposure to radioactivity, and then at this dosage for only a few weeks at a time. Iodine toxicity is possible. The RDA for iodine is 100mcg daily (one-tenth of a gram). Supplements such as Pacific Kelp (Lamberts) provide 150mcg per tablet, and thus the taking of ten of these would provide some 15 times the RDA. Is this reasonable or dangerous?

Ideal iodine intake

Professor Cheraskin, who conducted the successful trial enhancing defence against radiation damage in women receiving radiotherapy, described in the previous chapter, has studied this question. He analysed the iodine intake of over 1,000 doctors and found that the lowest intake was 100mcg and the highest 4.5gr, 4,500mcg, with an average intake for the whole group being 500mcg, some five times more than the RDA issued by the US Food and Nutrition Board.

He then provided these doctors with a questionnaire, which listed a total of 200 possible symptoms. These are either answered with a simple 'yes', if they suffered from such a symptom, or 'no' if not. The questionnaire (Cornell Medical Index) takes no more than ten minutes to complete. Analysis of the over 1,000 completed forms yielded the fact that the doctors with fewest symptoms noted were associated with a higher intake of iodine. The lower the iodine intake the more symptoms were noted on the questionnaire. The not unreasonable conclusion reached by Cheraskin was that the 'ideal' iodine intake, based on the evidence of these 1,000 healthy doctors, should be around 1,000mcg (1 mg) of iodine daily, which is ten times the RDA figure. He notes that in a number of similar trials he has consistently found that the ideal intake levels of most nutrients is always anything up to ten times greater than RDA.

Taking kelp for a short time, in quantities which provide sufficient alginate to accomplish the task of binding Strontium 90, would go beyond ten times RDA of iodine, and might reach 15 times this figure. It is therefore not suggested that this level of intake be maintained for more than a few weeks at a time, although unless there is evidence of iodine toxicity or allergy, an intake of ten times RDA would seem to be a positive health advantage.

Allergy too, or toxicity of iodine would display itself as a skin rash (such as acne), runny eyes, and/or nose, bronchitis and sore throat. Depression, insomnia and nervousness have been noted as well. Any such signs indicate an excess, and this may be remedied by reducing the dose until such symptoms stop. Allergy may, however, not stop until no kelp at all is being taken. This is unusual, and should lead to the adoption of other strategies outlined below. If allergy to iodine is noted it may still be possible to take pure alginate, which should be the first choice, if available, anyway. Evidence of the value of kelp in protecting against the effects of radioactivity is derived from a number of sources including the *International Journal of Radiation Biology*, 1971, pages 19 and 79-85. Also reference is found in *Medical World News* (7 March 1964) in an article by Dr R. Morgan, Chief Radiologist at John Hopkins University in America.

Pectin

Pectin is a fibre which is unlike most other fibres. It is soluble in hot water, and forms a gel when cooling, and is thus much used in cooking for the making of jelly-like dishes. It is found in many fruits and vegetables and is abundent in apples as well as sunflower seeds.

Its usefulness in an anti-radiation programme lies in the fact that it too binds Strontium 90 in the gastro-intestinal tract. If alginate is unavailable, or if there is sensitivity to kelp as a source, then pectin is recommended. Or both may be used alternately or in combination.

Pectin is available in tablet form from Larkhall Laboratories and also from Lamberts, in a form which combines it with acidophilus, itself a most desirable 'food' for the digestive system which helps to repopulate the bowel flora if this has been damaged. Acidophillus is discussed further later in the book.

The eating of several ounces of sunflower seeds daily and/or six apples a day, will provide ample pectin under moderately urgent conditions. However, if there has been exposure to radiation more may be needed. Mark Bricklin suggests: 'If you have access to apples, grate or mash two or three of them, and eat three or four times a day (6 to 12 apples a day). If using pectin tablets chew up and swallow a dozen of them, three or four times a day.'

The objective is to keep a presence of pectin in the bowel to work on any passing Strontium 90, which it will bind and carry with it out of the body. (Cooked apples are as useful as raw in providing pectin).

As Leslie Kenton points out in *Ageless Ageing* (Century Arrow, 1986) there are other advantages to be derived from its ingestion: 'Pectin appears to be an excellent substance for lowering cholesterol.' She continues: 'because of pectin's ability to bind cations and organic materials such as bile acids, it is also used as a natural chelating (binding) agent to take unwanted heavy metals such as aluminium in the system and to eliminate them from the body.'

Particularly rich sources of pectin are found in oranges, grapefruits, grapes and berries, as well as apples. It may be that an apple a day will not quite do what the old saying tells us, but half a dozen will help protect against radiation damage, as well as cholesterol excess, heavy metal toxicity etc.

When using pectin in this way additional vitamin C is suggested.

Evidence of the value of pectin in protection against radiation damage is noted in a number of references including *The Journal of the American Medical Association*, 18 November 1962, and in 'The Organic Consumer Report' of 8 August 1972 in an article by W. Baier (*Chemical Engineer*).

Bone meal, dolomite or calcium-magnesium supplementation

In the absence of either pectin or algin, or as an addition to their effective binding of radioactive elements in the system, the use is suggested of calcium and magnesium supplementation. Calcium, too, binds Strontium 90 in the bowel, and if there is an adequate calcium intake removes it from the system. Calcium has a natural affinity for some radioactive materials such as Strontium 90, which often finds its way into the bone structure in consequence.

If adequate calcium is provided as outlined below, then this will attract the circulating radioactive material, and will normally be eliminated from the system. Calcium is best combined with magnesium in supplementation. These are also of use in dealing with heavy metal toxicity, such as lead, mercury etc.

Bone meal is a powder commonly presented in tablet form, and is usually derived from the long bones of cattle. Its major constituent is calcium, together with some phosphorus and magnesium. These are in the same ratios as that found in human bones.

Dolomite is a mineral (limestone) and source of the elements calcium and magnesium in the ratio of two to one, which is the way the body handles them best. This too is found in health food stores in tablet form and either or both of these are the most reasonable way of obtaining adequate calcium and magnesium.

At least 1500mcg of calcium and 750mcg of magnesium are suggested as a daily intake, in dealing with existing radiation contamination or impending exposure. This will relieve to some extent the body of its burden of both radioactive Iodine

131 and Strontium 90. Again, as in the case of algin and pectin, the intake should be in split doses, at least four times daily, so that there is an ever present amount in the digestive tract.

Evidence of the value of bonemeal as a method of protecting against radiation is derived from research described in the National Cancer Institute's *Science Newsletter* of 2 March 1962.

Double Nobel prizewinner Linus Pauling discusses the value of calcium and magnesium in this regard, in *The New Yorker* ('These Precious Days') 3 October 1959. A bonus for anyone using a high vitamin C supplementation programme (as recommended) is that this will help the body to maintain heavy metals, including radioactive polonium (the radioactive element found in much tobacco smoke) in solution in the body, and thus allow them to be excreted via the urine.

Some forms of vitamin C are very acidic (when in the form of ascorbic acid or sodium ascorbate for example) and so it is suggested that a form be taken which enhances calcium intake, at the same time as providing ample vitamin C (the vitamin C part of these is the ascorbate). Calcium ascorbate is such a form, and is discussed in the section dealing with vitamin C. It is mentioned at this stage since it is a fine source of both ascorbate and calcium, and is a non-acid nutrient, which is desirable from the digestive tract's viewpoint. If this is unavailable then take vitamin C in any other form, and take powdered tablets or dolomite (calcium carbonate) at the same time, this will neutralize the acidity to some extent.

The strategies mentioned above may be used individually or in combination as deemed necessary in terms of the exposure to radiation in any given case. Algin and pectin are not too difficult to find. They may be taken as powders, tablets or directly from their natural sources, or in any combination of these.

Calcium and magnesium are available from natural sources (apples are very rich in calcium incidentally) as well as in tablet or powdered forms. Again these may be used in any combination as seems most appropriate and acceptable.

Vitamin C, which should always be part of an anti-radiation programme because of its antioxidant features, of which more later, is also useful as a means of direct excretion of toxic and radioactive metals. This bonus accompanies its prodigious use.

If we cannot avoid radiation then we can ensure that as much as possible is eliminated from the body. The substances mentioned above are all nutrients. The final substance discussed in this section is not, but is a safe, natural material.

Clay

Clay has well-known absorptive properties and is described in the *Dispensatory of the United States* as: 'In aqueous suspensions, the individual particles of clay (Bentonite) are negatively charged, thus resulting in a strong attraction for positively charged particles, and being responsible for it clarifying liquid, containing positively charged particles of suspended matter. In addition to the growing number of external uses for clay (Bentonite) it is reported to be of value as an intestinal evacuent when in the form of a gel.'

The absorbent powers of this substance are extraordinary. It has long been used to neutralize unpleasant smells, as well as toxic materials in healing.

Michael Abehsera points out (*The Healing Clay*, Swan House, 1978) that: 'Clay is particularly rich in certain diastases and enzymes, which do not destroy themselves in action. Some of these diastases, the oxidases, have the power of fixing free oxygen, which explains the purifying and enriching action of clay in the blood.'

Clay can absorb radioactivity. Abehsera tells us: 'On an organism which has suffered, and still retains the radiations of radium, or any other intensive radioactive source, the radioactivity... is absorbed.' This effect has been laboratory tested. Even dry clay is absorbent in this way. Clay has a unique structure in which its minute constituent particles, being rectangular, gives a large surface area in proportion to its volume, thus enabling it to pick up many more times than its own weight in positively charged particles. It is these positively charged particles which are the free radical enemies of the body. Radioactive materials are irresistibly drawn to clay (as they are to algin and pectin) where they are fixed and eventually eliminated from the body.

Since there is no absorption of clay there is no danger of the toxins once absorbed by the clay remaining in the body. Clay comes in a variety of forms. The French are devoted to green clay and the fine form of this (Argile vert surfine – fine green clay) is recommended for internal use. It may be taken in very small clay pellets, made by moistening the powder, then rolling it into pellets, and then baking these in an oven. Or it may be taken in suspension of water. If this method is chosen, and it is the simplest method, then the night before use, or at least several hours before, place a teaspoonful of fine green clay (French) into a half glass of spring water (unboiled). Stir and allow to settle.

At first consume just the water, leaving the residue. Later attempt to increase the amount of actual clay consumed in this manner (more of the teaspoon dose in the glass). Children should take half doses, and babies may be given a teaspoon of clay water before feeds. The normal time for taking clay is before breakfast, half an hour or so before eating.

If the drinking of the clay water, and some of its settled residue, is found difficult (although there is no particular taste it is slightly earthy) then the use of clay pellets, as mentioned, is suggested. It is also sometimes found to be more acceptable if mint, or another pleasant tasting herb, is used in the preparation of the paste, which is then baked into pellets. These may then be sucked instead of being swallowed.

Clay removes radioactive materials from the gut efficiently, and if there has been exposure to radioactivity, the dose, as mentioned above, can be doubled or trebled, so that a teaspoon of dissolved clay is consumed before each meal. In very rare cases there may be initial constipation, in which case liquid intake should be increased overall.

We have now examined safe methods for eliminating radioactive material from the body. The next consideration must be to minimize the effects of whatever radiation remains, and this calls, in a large part, for antioxidant action. We have looked in Chapter 2 at free radicals and how they work, as well as a brief survey of some of the anti-free-radical nutrients which exist. The next section will discuss these in detail, individually, with recommendation as to dosage etc.

5. The Free-Radical Scavengers And Quenchers

The single most important part of protecting the body against radiation damage, once radioactive material has entered the system, is the de-activation of free radical activity. This destructive oxidation of the body tissues requires anti-oxidants, free radical scavengers or quenchers, which will act to blot out the chain reaction of damage which these highly charged particles are capable of producing, and which lead to DNA (genetic material) alterations, which can end as cancer, as well as other cellular damage (see Chapter 2).

We will consider in a later section the methods and substances involved in enhancing the structural integrity of the cell membranes, and of promoting regeneration of damaged DNA. Some of the nutrients which are potent anti-oxidant, such as vitamin E, are involved in both free radical deactivation and cell membrane protection, and so will be mentioned in both sections.

In order to keep the types of nutrients discussed in this section in their family groups, vitamins, amino acids, etc. they will be so listed. This should not suggest a hierarchy of importance, however, since many of the nutrients active in antioxidant work interact with each other. This is essentially a team effort, and it should be understood that the use of only one or other of these nutrients, with no regard for the rest, is as futile as a football team fielding its best striker and perhaps its goalkeeper, and not bothering about the rest of the team, or perhaps just sending on the reserves.

The enemy in this battle for life itself is a fantastically well organized opponent, capable of a persistent and active process of destruction, and a full team is required to defend against this. Once started free radical destruction of cells can become a veritable chain reaction of damage which can get out of control. The main barrier to its continuation is the presence of the substances discussed below, the free radical fighters, the anti-oxidants.

We may divide the team of anti-oxidants into enzymes, amino acids, minerals and vitamins. There are also other substances which can beneficially influence the potential for damage, such as the adaptogens, such as ginseng and eleutherococcus, the actions of which will be explained after discussion of the individual elements of this defensive cohort of anti-oxidants and their supportive nutrients.

Enzyme anti-oxidants

One of the main substances involved in the body's defence against free radical activity is that most powerful of anti-oxidants, the enzyme *superoxide dismutase (SOD).*

There is a caution regarding the attempts which have been made to boost SOD activity by actual supplementation, which was sounded by the prestigious *American Journal of Clinical Nutrition*. This indicates that, whilst SOD in the body is indeed the best protection there is against such damage as may be triggered by the chain reaction of free radical action, the taking of SOD by mouth does not achieve the desired increase in its presence in the body. This failure to act relates to its molecular size, and its consequent inability to pass through the wall of the digestive tract into the body. For this reason SOD is not recommended for oral use, despite its obvious desirability. It would quite simply be a waste of money and effort, and until a method is found of ensuring SOD absorption this must remain a non-starter in a programme of defence against radiation and free radical damage. The elements which the body uses to manufacture SOD include the minerals zinc and copper, and these are, however, apparently capable of enhancing SOD production by the body.

A recent report in the *New Scientist* (12 June 1986) indicates that medical science is moving in this direction. Pharmacists at the University of Arkansas, have synthesized copper derivatives which induce protection against radiation damage. Mice given this copper were sufficiently protected for nearly 60 per cent of them to survive what was a lethal radiation dose. Moderate doses of organic copper and zinc are therefore desirable in promoting SOD-like reactions from cells challenged by radiation (see below for guidance as to dosage etc.)

It is the damaging potential of radiation which normally induces SOD production by cells. Overwhelmed by massive radiation and free radical activity, the SOD supply may be unable to cope, whether the source is X-ray therapy, a nuclear test or a Chernobyl-type disaster. The scavenging of free radical superoxides then falls to other defensive mechanisms.

The first line of defence in the body against the activity of free oxidizing radicals (FORs) are a series of enzymes which break them down. Of major importance in this role, as well as SOD, is the enzyme *glutathione peroxidase*. This is synthesized in the body from glutathione, an amino acid which will be discussed below, in combination with selenium which will also receive attention as we run through the antioxidant nutrients. The initial body response to FORs is for superoxide dismutase to de-activate the superoxide radical, into the less dangerous but still damaging form of hydrogen peroxide. This is further de-activated by a substance called catalase, or by glutathione peroxidase, by which it is returned to a harmless neutral state, such as water.

The superoxide free radical (O_2) is met and acted on by SOD to form a still dangerous substance – hydrogen peroxide (H_2O_2). If this then comes into contact with glutathione peroxidase or catalase it is de-activated to form water (H_2O). The taking of glutathione peroxidase as a supplement is not possible. Therefore its major ingredients need to be in plentiful supply and, as mentioned, these are selenium and glutathione. Superoxide dismutase is sold in health food stores, but remains controversial since its ability to be absorbed is debatable. In order to achieve adequate levels of SOD naturally in the body its co-factors need to be assured in the diet. These co-factors are zinc, copper and manganese.

Some evidence exists of increasing SOD activity via supplementation of these nutrients in forms which are bioavailable (i.e. easily abosorbed and transported by the body). Such forms exist as orotates or aspartates, which means that the minerals have been chelated (bound) to protein substances which are easily absorbed, and which, as it were, give the minerals a free ride into the body which they would find difficult to enter on their own.

Injectable forms of SOD exist, and these have been found useful in inflammatory athritis (animal trials) and could well prove of value in radiation damage conditions.

The measures whereby the activity of enzymes against FORs are activated therefore seem to depend, at least in part, upon the ample presence in the system of minerals and amino acids, which will be discussed in this section, since apart from the injectable form of SOD which remains experimental, and the oral form which remains of questionable value, the body has to make its own protective enzymes.

The body responds to the stress of exposure to free radical damage by producing increased levels of protective enzymes. This is thought by some initially to have a generally beneficial effect on the organism, and produces the apparent paradox of a little exposure to smog or radiation, for example, being a desirable thing. However, once the exposure goes beyond a mild increase the additional free radical activity overwhelms the increased enzyme presence, and destruction of tissues commences. Also, the dubious benefits which such exposure might produce depend very much on the adequacy of the body in producing the appropriate defensive enzymes, which is itself dependent upon nutrients such as zinc and copper being present. These are the frontline soldiers against FORs, and they need to be supported by every means safely achievable. So should the amino acids which are part of the second line of defence.

Amino acids

Amino acids are the building material of protein; our bodies requiring twenty-two of these with which to construct the materials of our various component tissues. All, apart from eight of these amino acids, can be produced in the body from other material. These eight, however, have to be present in our food, at the same time and in the correct proportions, for the synthesis of protein to be adequate to the needs of health maintenance.

It is often asked why there should be any need for the supplementation of individual amino acids if adequate protein is being eaten. The answer lies in the structure of protein in food, in which long chains of amino acids are present. In order for these to be of any use to the body they need to be broken down into their individual constituent amino acids. This is often not achieved because of enzyme deficiencies and an imbalanced diet. The form in which amino acids are provided in supplements is known as 'free form'. This means that the amino acids are ready for use immediately.

Many roles have been discovered for the different amino acids. Some are used therapeutically to great advantage, and since they are part of the natural economy of the body they tend to be less toxic than artificial drugs. Caution should be exercised, however, since, as with all things, there can be harmful effects if used wrongly under certain conditions.

The major amino acid support against FORs is from a triple amino acid compound called *glutathione*. This is made up of three amino acids and is thus called a tripeptide. The constituents of this are cysteine, glutamine and glycine. Whereas glutathione acts against free radicals outside the cells of the body, the activity of glutathione peroxidase is largely intracellular. There is a great deal of evidence of the protective value of this safe amino acid compound, ranging from protection against cancer development, heavy metal detoxification, retarding of ageing process, and increased liver detoxification activity (against alcohol for example).

It also acts to increase the effectiveness of vitamin C in its antioxidant and detoxification roles. A dosage of between one and three grams daily of glutathione is suggested for its detoxification and protective role against free radical activity if there has been exposure to radiation. The doses should be taken with water, not a protein drink such as milk, and at least half an hour before meals. One of the components of glutathione, the sulphur-containing amino acid *cysteine*, is a powerful antioxidant and detoxification agent, in its own right. It binds to dangerous free radical particles rendering them harmless. When combined with vitamins C and B_1, cysteine protects cells from the damaging effects of radiation (as well as other toxic substances). It is important not to confuse cysteine with cystine, another amino acid.

Cysteine is recommended for all chronic forms of ill health, where dosages of 3g a day (taken in three separate 1g doses) for a month, followed by a reduction for a month to 2g daily, and then a maintenance dose of 1g daily, are prescribed. It should be taken with vitamin B_6, in doses of 50mg for each 1g of cysteine, as this helps in its activation. In order to prevent cysteine's conversion to cystine it should be taken with vitamin C (three times the amount of C to cysteine). Caution should be exercised by diabetics in whom cysteine might cause problems since it de-activates insulin to a certain extent.

As will be noted later, vitamins C and B_6 are a part of the anti-radiation programme, and the use of cysteine could well accompany this in addition to, or instead of glutathione, of which it is an integral part.

Russian cosmonauts use a complex of vitamins and amino acids in order to protect against the harmful effects of radiation and stress. Amongst the ingredients of this complex are two amino acids tryptophan and histidine. The presence of *tryptophan* in an anti-radiation package is puzzling since it has no anti-oxidant or anti-radiation capabilities. However, its role in mood alteration is well known, and this may well be why the Russians have included it. Also, tryptophan is valuable as an antidepressant and as a relaxant prior to sleep (together with vitamin B_6 and magnesium). A derivative of tryptophan in the body, is the important neurotransmitter serotonin, and this is the clue to tryptophan's usefulness in a variety of mental and emotional problems. Dietary sources of tryptophan are often limited since it is not plentiful in food and what little there is can be destroyed in cooking.

Histidine on the other hand is an interesting amino acid which has been used effectively in treating rheumatoid arthritis. In this regard it is thought to help by removal of heavy metal contamination (copper for example) which might be aggravating the condition. Its ability to chelate metals is one reason for its possible value in radiation exposure. It is the precursor of histamine, and is thus involved in a number of allergic conditions as well as being a major element in sexual arousal.

Histidine is reported to be necessary for the maintenance of the myelin sheath of the nerves, and this is a probable area in which it is useful against the effects of radiation. In the first overwhelming wave of radiation it is the nervous system which is most damaged. Protection against this is apparently one beneficial role which histidine is thought to offer. Therefore it should be thought of as a protective element rather than one to use after exposure. The Russian cosmonauts take their protective mixture, including histadine, some fifteen minutes prior to anticipated exposure. This could well be a strategy to follow for those having radiotherapy.

The Russian amino acid-vitamin mix includes vitamins B_1, B_6, bioflavonoids, vitamin C, histidine, tryptophan and some trace elements such as selenium and zinc. They also use the adaptogen ginseng. Histidine is not, however, an antioxidant as such (apart from its ability to remove heavy metals which would promote free radical activity further) and its role in anti-radiation protection depends upon less specific activities.

Dosages commonly suggested for tryptophan and histidine are as follows:

Tryptophan for general usage, 300mg daily. For sleep enhancement, 1g together with vitamin B_6, vitamin C and magnesium prior to sleep. For depression, 3g daily plus 1g of vitamin B_3 (niacinamide).

Histidine for heavy metal removal, 6g daily together with

vitamin C. Histidine should be used with caution by anyone who is a manic depressive, since some such individuals have excessive levels of histamine in the body.

Taurine is another amino acid used in free radical control. Its main benefits in this area (it has a variety of other roles in the body) resulting from its unique ability to neutralize the ionic form of chlorine (hypochlorite). It also regulates intracellular calcium levels which is of some importance in radiation exposure. Taurine is directly related to the levels of zinc in the blood. Dosage of between 100mg and 1g daily are used at first, reducing to as little as 50mg daily.

In a specific attempt to minimize radiation damage, glutathione and cysteine should be used. Histidine is thought to be of protective value only rather than of use after the event. This could be combined with the other nutrients mentioned above if this protective strategy is being attempted (note vitamin E's role in protecting against radiation damage as discussed in Chapter 3).

The amino acids are vital in their role as anti-oxidants and as precursors of the enzymes discussed at the beginning of this chapter.

Vitamins

We will now look at the marvellous protective qualities of the vitamins before going on to consider minerals and other substances.

Vitamin A. This fat-soluble vitamin is a powerful anti-oxidant as well as having specific effects which defend cell structures. It occurs in two forms, the vitamin itself, or its precursor *beta carotene*, from which the body makes its own vitamin A. Both forms are anti-oxidants. Vitamin A's main area of activity is in protecting the vital epithelial linings of the intestinal tract, the lungs and the mucous membranes generally. It has been found that cells which have become altered and precancerous, are with vitamin A activity, capable of recovery and of regaining normality.

The more of the other anti-oxidants that are being consumed (vitamins C, E etc.) the less vitaminA is required over and above the body's normal requirements, but its antioxidant role as a free radical quencher is vital in protecting the tissues mentioned.

In any nutrient supplementation there is a most important and often neglected element, and that is bioavailability. The taking of a nutrient supplement is not enough. It has to be absorbed and transported to its desired site before the body can use it. In considering fat-soluble vitamins in particular (as well as certain minerals) there are often problems associated with absorption and use by the body. Fat-soluble vitamins such as vitamin A are dependent upon the efficiency of a complex range of digestive processes. By copying the method used by the human mother (providing fat-soluble vitamin A in a water-soluble form in mother's milk) some manufacturers have been able to enhance absorption and bioavailability of this important nutrient. Sources exist of water-soluble vitamin A and E (see page 88). A dose of 20,000 to 25,000iu daily of vitamin A, in this form, is suggested in an anti-radiation programme. Toxicity may occur if doses of 100,000iu or more are taken for long periods. In infants a maximum level of 15,000iu daily is suggested.

Any side-effects of over-dosage (flaking of the skin, nausea, hair loss, headache, fatigue and liver enlargement) will disappear with reduction of dosage to normal levels. Overdosage is unnecessary, though, since the moderate intakes recommended are suitable for all those also taking other antioxidants. Taking the beta carotene precursor of vitamin A is entirely non-toxic, however. Since only some of this substance is converted into vitamin A, and the rest circulates in the blood and acts as an antioxidant factor, it is of value in an anti-radiation programme. In addition to 20,000 to 25,000iu of water-miscible vitamin A being taken, about 25mg of beta carotene is a useful addition to the defence system.

Vitamin B complex. A number of nutrient substances related chemically to each other are grouped into the B complex. Some of these are vitally involved in anti-radiation activity. These include vitamins B_1, B_5, and B_6. We will examine these individually since they play different roles.

Vitamin B_1 (thiamine). This water-soluble nutrient is intimately involved in the process which produces energy in the body, as well as being involved in the manufacture of acetyl choline which is vital for nerve function, among other important roles. It is an anti-oxidant factor and as such works with other elements towards this protective end.

Together with vitamin C and the sulphur-rich amino acid cysteine, it protects against dangerous free-radical-producing substances, and reduces the chances of cross-linkage damage in tissues. In order that the taking of this nutrient should not disturb the biochemical balance of the body it should be accompanied by all other vitamin B substances.

In a manner similar to that indicated for the substances which bind to radioactive material in the digestive tract (pectin etc.) there should be a divided dosage of anti-free radical substances, which are water soluble. Vitamin B_1 is eliminated from the body fairly quickly if it is surplus to tissue requirements. Thus a steady supply is desirable during the day when radiation is a problem and defence is required. Three or four divided doses during the day will do far more good than will one large dose. The quantity suggested is of three or four 25mg to 50mg doses daily, together with other B vitamins, vitamin C and cysteine, if possible.

Vitamin B_5, (pantothenic acid) in the form of calcium pantothenate). This is important in the function of the adrenal gland. It has multiple roles in the body of which many relate to defence against stress-induced damage, especially of the nerve structures. It, too, is vital to the conversion of other substances, such as choline (see below) to acetylcholine in the brain, where it is a vital neurotransmitter. Vitamin B_5 slows down or prevents cross-linkage tissue damage, which is so much a part of free radical activity after radiation exposure. It also enhances the immune (defence) function of the body. It, too, should be taken in divided doses. As with thiamine, toxic levels are virtually unheard of, and three to four doses of between 25mg and 100mg daily are suggested as part of an anti-radiation strategy, together with other B-vitamins.

It is always wise to begin taking such nutrients at the lower levels advised, and to build up to the higher levels of intake so that tolerance is increased. A sudden intake of high dosages can produce diarrhoea and other reactions. These are less likely when care is taken over introduction.

Vitamin B_6 (pyridoxine). As previously mentioned this is a very important nutrient indeed. It is a constituent part of a great many hormones and enzymes, without which body functions would virtually cease. It is a major part of the immune function as well as being involved in the digestion of fats, proteins and carbohydrates. Adequate amounts in the body are necessary for DNA and RNA to be manufactured. As noted, it is used by many radiologists to prevent or treat the symptoms of nausea, which often accompany radiotherapy. It also stops cross-linkage damage in tissues threatened by free radical activity.

A high intake of meat causes an increased body need for B_6, as does alcohol intake, smoking, the birth control pill, etc. It is also needed for the conversion of histidine to histamine, and without the correct balance sexual function can become impaired. It is important that when taking B_6 and equal amount of vitamin B_2 (riboflavin) be taken in order to prevent biochemical imbalances from occurring in the body.

Toxicity has been reported when doses reach several thousand milligrams daily, but there is no need for such high doses to be attempted. Being a water-soluble nutrient, as are all other B vitamins, it should be taken in divided doses during the day. Quantities of 50mg to 100mg three times daily should be taken as part of a radiation protection programme.

Thus we have three of the B vitamins which require divided dosages, as well as at least one other (B_2), which needs to be taken in order to maintain biochemical balance. The suggested strategy is to obtain from a reliable source (see page 88) a high strength B-complex formula, which contains at least 25mg and ideally 100mg each of B_1, B_2, B_6 and calcium pantothenate (which may be listed as B_5). If the constituents listed above are present in 25mg doses then take three or four of the B-complex tablets or capsules daily with or after food. If the ingredients are in 50mg or 100mg doses then take a half or a quarter tablet four times daily for a week, before increasing gradually to a level of four full strength tablets daily, containing 100mg each of these B vitamins. By taking the whole complex rather than individual tablets of B_1, B_5, B_6 etc. a great deal of bother is prevented and, more importantly, the balance between B vitamins is constantly maintained. The colour of the urine will alter when these doses of B vitamins are taken. This is quite normal, and has no sinister significance. Anything from a bright yellow to a greenish hue will be noted.

Another way of taking B vitamins is to use Brewer's yeast in powder or tablet form and to take this in very large amounts. Russian research (D-kl. Akad. Nauk. SSDR Bd. 126, p 417) indicates that brewer's yeast has a strong radiation protection effect. It certainly contains the B vitamins in good balance, and so can be seen as a cheaper way of obtaining them. At least three tablespoonfuls of yeast powder (or 12 to 15 tablets) daily would be needed to achieve reasonable levels of B vitamin intake.

Note: A caution is needed for people with problems related to yeast sensitivity or allergy. There are yeast-free sources of B vitamins (see page 90) and these should be used where symptoms of bloatedness, nausea, dizziness or other side-effects are noted when yeast is ingested. In such cases my book *Candida Albicans: Could Yeast Be Your Problem?* (Thorsons, 1985) should be looked at for advice on simple methods of improving this situation.

The B vitamins listed are not major anti-oxidants in themselves, but they support the efforts of other nutrients. They are so vital in the defence of the body generally that the importance of their presence in a programme designed to protect against radiation damage cannot be over-emphasized.

Vitamin C. This is a major anti-oxidant and defender of cell integrity. Many millions of years ago cosmic radiation appears to have destroyed in man the ability to manufacture the substance ascorbate. All (or almost all) other animals have retained this ability. In evolutionary terms, it is thought by researchers that the loss of this manufacturing ability was initially an advantage. Living at that time in lush tropical forest with an abundance of green plants and fresh fruits within easy reach there was no disadvantage to early man in nutritional terms. All the vitamin C he needed was near to hand, as it still is today for the mountain gorilla, for example. The release of the machinery for the internal manufacture of this vitamin was an advantage in that it freed the body from energy and effort which could then be used elsewhere. Experiments on tiny, fast-breeding creatures such as fruit flies, shows that when a genetic alteration is engineered which releases some of them from the need to perform a particular biochemical task, these experimental creatures end up dominant in groups where they are mixed with identical creatures which still have to perform particular internal manufacturing tasks, such as the synthesis of an enzyme or vitamin etc.

This evolutionary advantage in man became a disadvantage, however, when he was forced by climatic changes to leave his forest fastnesses and take to hunting and gathering in order to survive. There was no way of switching the genetic machinery on again and man requires a constant intake of ascorbate in order to survive. Unfortunately he does not get adequate amounts, since the fresh fruits and fresh vegetables currently eaten in the industrialized world is low in comparison to the real needs of the body.

As far as radiation protection is concerned vitamin C is one of the most important, if not the most important, requirements. This relates to its powerful anti-oxidant qualities as well as its integral part in the intercellular structures of the body. It thus protects and binds the material of the body and is irreplacable in anti-radiation defence.

Some studies indicate that we need between 500mg and 2,500 mg of vitamin C daily, but official RDAs tend to be much lower because health authorities base their recommendations on the amounts necessary to avoid signs of obvious deficiency. Thus around 60mg to 80mg daily is suggested. There is, though, strong evidence pointing to a far greater need.

All stress factors destroy, or use up, vitamin C in the body, at a very fast rate indeed. Where it is operating in its anti-oxidant and cell-protecting role the body's requirement is even higher. Is there a way of finding out our requirements, under any particular condition? Thankfully, the answer is yes. There are at least two simple ways of doing this:

1. A simple test kit is available from Larkhall Laboratories (see page 87). This requires that a drop of purple solution be placed on the tongue whilst a watch is kept on the time it takes

to disappear. This indicates accurately the current adequacy or otherwise of vitamin C status. If it takes longer than it should (all details are on the pack) then more vitamin C is needed in the body. By taking a dose and retesting later the adequacy of this is assessed and eventually we can reach a point where the colour placed on the tongue vanishes quickly, indicating that the body is well loaded with vitamin C. This can be a laborious business, but is a useful and accurate guide to the body's status of this vital nutrient.

2. The method of choice is to load the body with vitamin C in ever increasing amounts until it tells you to stop. This is done by beginning an intake of 2g or 3g per day of vitamin C, in divided doses (vitamin C is a water-soluble substance and is not stored in any quantity, thus a constant supply is needed). The dosage should be increased by a gram per day until eventually a mild diarrhoea is noted (or a degree of flatulence). At this level of intake the body is 'saturated', and intake should be reduced to the level of vitamin C taken the previous day, where no such symptoms were noted. The symptoms will rapidly disappear and should cause no alarm; they simply indicate that the body is eliminating the excessive amounts.

Such a method could of course take a week or more to reach the point where optimum amounts are being taken to meet current needs. A variation on this method is to begin high dosage immediately when there is a need for additional vitamin C (extreme stress, infection of any sort, exposure to radiation etc.) For instance, 1g to 2g every two hours can be taken. This might well trigger a response of diarrhoea which will soon pass if the intake is meeting the needs of the body.

Many people, because of their own biochemical individuality, actually function best on intakes of 10g to 15g of vitamin C all the time. Others only need a dosage of 2g to 3g under conditions of stress or illness, and function well on daily doses of half a gram or less under normal conditions.

Whenever very high doses of vitamin C have been taken, the return to a normal maintenance dose of between 500mg to 2g daily should be made step by step. Thus, if 10g per day is being taken due to exposure to radiation, or to some illness, then reduction afterwards should be by a gram a day until the maintenance amount is reached. This avoids a rebound effect which can occur when there is a sudden cessation of a high intake.

The antioxidant effects of vitamin C cannot be over-emphasized, and this is one of its key roles in radiation protection.

There are many forms of vitamin C, and the cheapest is as a powder or crystal which can be dissolved in water or juice and consumed at regular intervals through the day (see page 88 for sources). If a less acid form is required, then calcium ascorbate should be used in powder or tablet form. The level of well-being and improved overall function, which a high dosage of this marvellous substance can produce, needs to be experienced to be believed. No toxic effects are to be anticipated, despite the grossly exaggerated claims of some detractors that kidney stones might develop (they actually are less likely than ever on a high vitamin C intake, especially if vitamin B_6 and magnesium are adequately present, as they would be in the anti-radiation programme) or that vitamin B_{12} might be destroyed with high vitamin C intake. This has been shown to be a false claim. There are no dangers, only benefits.

Intake is suggested of not less than 5g daily if radiation exposure is suspected or anticipated. Vitamin C is one of the nutrients used in Russian space travel radiation protection, and this is taken before anticipated radiation exposure. Thus anyone having radiotherapy could well include a dose, together with other appropriate nutrients before exposure.

In nature vitamin C is usually found in combination with a range of substances called *bioflavonoids*. These are a major element in radiation protection. The relationship between vitamin C and these is so close that they have been dubbed 'vitamin C complex.' Their role in this programme is as cell protectors in both an anti-oxidant role and a cell membrane stabilizer.

Quercitin is a flavonoid which is present in many plants and is known to have strong anti-inflammatory and cell protective abilities. It is used in many inflammatory processes and allergic conditions to good effect, and is just one example of the many other flavonoids which are present in plants. These include *hesperidin, rutin, nobiletin* etc. They are often grouped together under the same name of vitamin P, and are frequently incorporated into vitamin C formulations. They may be taken separately in dosages of a gram a day or more, in divided doses, or in combination with vitamin C. These too are part of the Russian formula against radiation.

Vitamin E. This is the most powerful anti-oxidant and, indeed, it is suggested by many that this is its sole role in the body. Vitamin E is a fat-based vitamin and therefore can be stored in the body. It comes in a variety of forms and it is important when purchasing a vitamin E supplement to ensure that it is *d-alpha tocopherol* which is being bought. There is a vast amount of research evidence which points to the protective regenerative role of Vitamin E where oxidation has produced cell damage. This is as true in the bone marrow as it is in the liver or the intestinal tract.

With the World Health Organization estimating that 75 per cent of all human cancers are caused by environmental factors, and other researchers showing that as much as 90 per cent of cancers may be thus induced, the potential role of vitamin E as a protective agent is profound. Most of the environmental agents which produce, or induce, cell changes and which end as cancer, involve oxidation and peroxidation, much of this deriving from free radical activity. The sources of this damaging oxidation are many, including undesirable dietary patterns, but having as a major element ionizing radiation (as well as ultra-violet radiation) which generate free radicals in the body. Even when the cells of the body have become pre-cancerous and have a high mitotic index (i.e. they are dividing rapidly and are almost out of control) vitamin E has been able to induce regeneration of normal function and structure.

At least 1,000iu of vitamin E (d=alpha tocopherol) should be taken daily in an anti-radiation programme, and the ideal form of this is (as in the case of vitamin A) a water-miscible one. This ensures ease of absorption which a fat soluble vitamin requires in the human system. It has been shown that the normal fat based forms of vitamin E are poorly absorbed and that water-miscible forms (see page 88) are infinitely better handled by the body.

Minerals and trace elements

We have previously noted that *selenium* is an important factor in protecting the body against cancer and heart disease. It accomplishes these tasks by being an anti-oxidant, a component of glutathione peroxidase, and also by interacting synergistically with vitamin E. This latter observation means that on its own it does something good, as does vitamin E. Together they do more than the sum of their individual efforts would indicate possible. We must ensure that as well as vitamin E we are also able to obtain a good source of selenium in an anti-radiation programme.

Recall that as part of glutathione peroxidase, selenium will be protecting the cell membrances against oxidative damage. Cell membrane damage followed by disruption of genetic material and consequent mutation are the most damaging effects of radiation, and this protection offered by the selenium compound glutathione peroxidase is a critical one. It is in this way that heart disease and cancer are protected against, since free radical oxidative damage often leads on to these chronic problems. The starting point of cancer and of most cardiovascular disease is in free radical damage to tissues.

Selenium may be toxic if taken excessively, and so the recommendation is for no more than 400mcg daily being taken, in divided doses to aid absorption.

The final elements which we will be looking at in this section on anti-free radical agents are *zinc* and *copper*. Neither are strictly speaking anti-oxidants. They are, however, a vital part of that most potent of all anti-oxidants, superoxide dismutase (SOD). There is evidence of zinc being a major element in slowing cross-linkage damage in tissues, and in being a powerful wound healing agent. These abilities may relate to increased SOD presence, with zinc supplementation. Certain forms of cancer are known to increase when zinc is deficient and, again, this may relate to SOD inadequacy resulting from low zinc levels. Zinc works in many body processes with vitamin B_6 which, as we have seen, has a primary role in reducing the symptoms of radiation damage. For a variety of reasons, therefore, zinc is incorporated into a programme of anti-radiation protection. Dosages of 15mg to 50mg daily are suggested in the form of zinc orotate. This form ensures any easy uptake by the body of what might otherwise pass through the digestive tract unabsorbed. When zinc orotate is taken the individual tablets will state 200mg of B_{13} zinc (B_{13} is the tentative symbol for orotic acid). The actual amount of zinc in such a formulation will be around 15mg, the rest being the orotate with which it is bound for ease of absorption.

Copper and zinc are actually antagonistic in that they fight for absorption by the body. Therefore, they should not be taken at the same time. A useful strategy, if supplementation of both is undertaken, is to take zinc for three days of the week and copper orotate (B_{13} copper) for one. Continuing this alternation allows for absorption of both and consequent enhancement of SOD activity, SOD depends upon both nutrients in body tissues. A dose of 10mg of B_{13} copper is therefore suggested, on a rotation basis, with zinc orotate, as described above.

To summarize the approach to anti-radiation damage control in the body as far as free radical activity is concerned:

Amino acids cysteine and glutathione are essential (cysteine with vitamin B_6 and vitamin C).

Histidine may be employed in a protective role if radiation exposure is anticipated.

Vitamins A (and beta carotene) in modest doses as described.

Vitamin C (and bioflavonoids) in high doses as described.

Vitamin E is essential in radiation protection, but not with breast cancer.

B complex (B_1, B_5 and B_6 specifically, or large yeast intakes) as well as selenium, should always be a part of this programme.

Copper and zinc, both in orotate form, in dosages as outlined above.

All dosages should vary with the degree of exposure. the forms of the nutrients are important, and water-miscible vitamins A and E are desirable for ease of absorption. B vitamins should be combined as outlined, and vitamin C should be stepped up until adequate saturation of tissues is achieved. Cysteine and glutathione should be taken away from other foods, to ensure lack of competition in the digestive system, as well as ease of absorption.

6. Protection And Regeneration Of The Body Cell Membranes And DNA

We have now looked at what initial nutritional defences there are against radiation, involving attempts to eliminate radioactive material from the system and to control the spread of free oxidizing radicals. The next step is to review ways by which we can reduce cell membrane damage, reduce and repair DNA and RNA damage and, overall, minimize radiation effects. The substances involved in such strategies are to some extent the same as those involved in free radical scavenging and anti-oxidant activity, with some additional ones. We will first be considering aspects of the protective roles of the adaptogens ginseng and eleutherococcus, as well as pollen and royal jelly, and other useful nutrients and substances.

What is an adaptogen?

Put very simply it is a substance which helps the body to adapt successfully and without any harmful effects in order to cope with stress. To qualify as an adaptogen it should have protective properties of a general nature, thus enhancing a wide range of functions and protecting against a wide variety of potentially harmful factors. In saying that its effects should be non-specific, it is meant that, unlike many substances which have specific effects (painkiller, tranquillizer etc.) adaptogens should be able to enhance the body's own recuperative powers (also called homeostasis; describing the balancing, normalizing functions of the body) whatever the nature of the problem. Adaptogens should therefore be able to help protect against the damaging effects of radiation, whatever these might involve.

Reactive free radicals in the tissues of the body cumulatively disturb and clog the metabolic machinery. The proteins of the cells become cross-linked and aged. The structure of protein is coded in the genetic material DNA (desoxyribonucleic acid) and the information as to cell construction is carried to building sites by ribonucleic acid (RNA). Sometimes, as the result of free radical damage, often resulting from radiation, this vital reproductive mechanism becomes imperfect. The RNA carrying its blueprint instructions may become defective resulting in cell building abberations. These aberrant cells will not function quite as well as they should, and eventually cell damage repair may become so imperfect that functions are altered. Ageing will have taken place, sometimes long before time would have accomplished the same effect.

If animals are mildly irradiated experimentally (with X-rays) their lifespan becomes shortened in proportion to the amount of radiation used, and this is directly parallel to the observable damage to the DNA/RNA structures caused by the radiation. Sometimes, of course, more damage than the mild general decline in function outlined above occurs, and mutant cells become uncontrolled in their replication. Cancer will have developed. When and how often this occurs relates directly to the nutritional status of the tissues of the animal, or the person, thus exposed. This is where optimum levels of the nutrients already discussed in previous chapters can be shown to act as life preservers and cancer inhibitors. Adaptogens should be able to protect against this sort of damage as well. Can they? It appears so.

Ginseng is an adaptogen of amazing antiquity having been used in the Orient for thousands of years as a substance which prolongs the active period of life. Russian trials on animals have shown that ginseng can prolong the life of experimental rats by about 15 per cent.

Eleutherococcus is a Siberian plant which is similar to, and apparently more powerful than, ginseng. It raised the lifespan of rats by 16.5 per cent and is known to be a powerful anti-oxidant. Endurance is enhanced and, as would be anticipated from an adaptogen, it reduces the effect of all types of stress, without causing any side-effects.

Russian scientists, investigating anti-radiation methods, give prime place to these two adaptogens, ginseng and eleutherococcus, since they increased resistance more profoundly, to a wider range of unfavourable effects, whether these be chemical, physical or biological, than any other substance studied.

Brekhman, in his book *Man and Biologically Active Substances* (Pergamon Press, 1980) tells of experiments where mice were subjected to highly toxic substances and in which high doses of ginseng and eleutherococcus were able to offer protection to an amazing degree. Of all the adaptogens studied, eleutherococcus is found to be the most effective and to be harmless to the body.

Professor Roger Williams, (University of Texas), discoverer of pantothenic acid (vitamin B_5) found that it increased the lifespan of experimental animals by about 15 per cent, retarding the general decline in the quality of cell structure and DNA replication considerably.

One of the best sources of pantothenic acid is *royal jelly*, the material which is given to the queen bee by its colony. Secreted by the worker bees, royal jelly contains almost all nutrients known. Bulgarian research has shown its usefulness in radiation protection. Leslie Kenton states: 'They (the Bulgarians) have found for instance that royal jelly has an ability to protect against radiation.' It does a number of other amazing things, and is in every way a desirable addition to health promotion. It may be termed adaptogen, since it reduces the effects of stress and enhances health with no harmful effects. Sources of these adaptogens are given on page 89.

Pollen is another non-specific nutrient source, which also shows itself capable of offering protection against the effects of radiation. As mentioned earlier, pollen has been used in both cancer patients and animals, receiving radiation, and has proved protective.

There is no way at present of knowing whether these effects relate to nutrients such as those discussed in the previous chapter, which might be present in pollen or royal jelly, or whether there are other substances in them, acting in a beneficial manner. The benefits of pollen may relate to its general adaptogen function, or indeed to its content of nutrients, or to both. Essential fatty acids, which will be discussed later, are plentiful in pollen, and this may be the reason for its well documented protective role in radiation exposure.

With any adaptogen it is necessary to take the substance regularly and for some time before a noticeable effect is produced. A gram or two daily of ginseng or eleutherococcus is suggested, and a month or more should be anticipated before benefits are felt. With radiation damage this is obviously a long time to wait, and so the regular use of such substances in everyday life as non-specific protective agents is indicated.

Ignoring the powerhouse of activity which is continuous in all body cells, the outer envelope within which the life of the cell is carried out, is called the cell membrance. This is constructed in the main from special fats and lipids. It must be not only strong but capable of allowing the selective passage into the cell of the nutrients required by them, as well as oxygen for respiration, and also the passage outwards of waste materials.

In a way each cell is a miniature creature, with a function of its own and the ability, usually, to reproduce itself exactly. Once there is damage to the membrane of the cell, or of the membranes of the minute structures within the cell which have individual functions such as protein synthesis and waste disposal, there is disruption of function. The waste materials which should be extruded from the cell may contaminate it and poison it; protein may be mis-synthesized, and in general the cell will cease to function normally.

The cell membranes are, therefore, more important than mere coverings, they are the protectors of the vital processes which go on inside them, as well as actually being a functional material in allowing passage, on a selective basis, of materials into or out of the cell. Free radical activity damages the membrane more easily than other tissues since it is largely comprised of fatty cells, which are vulnerable to peroxidation.

Essential fatty acids

The type of fats which play the major part in the construction of cell membranes are called *essential fatty acids (EFA)*. Just as some amino acids were 'essential', inasmuch as they could not be synthesized by the body, so fatty acids are essential when they must be provided in the diet. EFAs are also a component of the materials which bind cells together to give tissue cohesion. They are divided into different groups based on their structure and function.

Linolenic acid, from which is made *gamma linolenic acid (GLA)*, belongs to what is called the omega 6 group of EFAs. A second group is the omega 3 family of EFAs, which has as its major constituent *alpha linolenic acid* and from this are derived other substances including *eicosapentaenoic acid (EPA) and docosahexaenoic acid (DHA).* It is from these that cell membrane structures are constructed, as well as their having a wide range of other roles to play in the body's economy. Whilst it is possible, through the diet, to obtain all these EFAs adequately, there are times when supplementation is desirable to ensure that the right types of EFAs are entering the system. About 4 to 6 capsules, each containing 500mg of EFAs, are recommended.

Such substances as *linseed oil, Evening Primrose oil* and individual EFA derivatives such as the fish body extract *max-EPA* are all useful methods of obtaining a supply of these nutrients, where cell membrane damage has occurred or might occur.

Dietary sources are from seeds (such as sunflower, sesame, linseed, pumpkin etc.) all of which are available in health food stores. Other sources are oily fish such as mackerel and herring.

The B vitamins *inositol and choline* are cell membrane stabilizers as is another B vitamin derivative *PABA (para amino benzoic acid)*. Vitamin E plays a similar protective role for the cell membranes, as does zinc. We have previously discussed *zinc, vitamins E, C and the bioflavonoids* (which have a particularly strong influence in this area of protection) and so should give a little attention to those nutrients which we have not discussed, inositol, choline and PABA.

Both inositol and choline should form a part of any vitamin B complex which is being taken (as a source of B_1, B_5, B_6 etc. as advised in the previous chapter) and so the adequacy of their intake should be assured. These B-complex tablets commonly contain 50mg to 100mg each of choline and inositol, and with three to four B-complex tablets required for a radiation protection programme this would supply between 200mg and 400mg each day of each of these two vitamins. This is the lowest level of intake desirable, and additional supplementation could be achieved by the taking of choline and inositol individually, as well, in order to reach a minimum intake of 750mg to 1,000mg daily in actual radiation exposure situations.

PABA is also frequently found in B-complex tablets, and a dosage of 250mg to 500mg should be taken in any effort to ensure cell membrane stabilization.

If the nutrients described in Chapter 5 are being used as outlined, then the additional use of EFAs as described above, with attention paid to obtaining extra choline, inositol and PABA will accomplish as much protection as is possible from damage to cell membranes. Vitamin E in particular is a major defender of these tissues and, together with the vitamin C-bioflavonoid defence, permits as far as possible protection against cell membrane destruction and the consequences of this.

The repair of mis-synthesized components of protein in cellular structures is accomplished by the use of the amino acids described in previous chapters, *cysteine,* and *glutathione*. Their *sulphur* and *selenium* component encourages normalization of such damaged proteins as are found in cells injured by free radical attack. Cysteine and glutathione, together with the additional selenium being taken, as described previously, offer the best opportunity for normalizing such damage. Foods which provide rich amounts of sulphur, and which are protective, are: cabbage, garlic, onions and eggs. Selenium is found in eggs, onions, garlic (very rich), brewer's yeast, wheat germ, cabbage and tomatoes. The best sources of vitamin E, which is so involved in these defensive actions are wheat germ, leafy vegetables, eggs, fish, whole grains and vegetable oils.

It can be seen from the above that onions, garlic, eggs and the brassica family are all highly desirable foods, as are all green leafy vegetables.

Nucleic acid therapy

We have previously looked at amino acids and their importance in the body. The construction of proteins in the body from these individual amino acids depends upon RNA being present in sufficient quantities. Whereas DNA provides the genetic message as to what form the construction should take, it is RNA which carries that message. Absence of the adequate RNA prevents protein synthesis. Thus the provision of the raw materials from which RNA is constructed is a logical aim in restoration of function such as protein synthesis, without which the body cannot survive.

Once damaged it is though that regeneration of DNA is possible, and there is evidence of vitamin A and E influencing such a return to normal in aberrant cells (see previous chapters). American and German research has laid the foundation for another approach – Nucleic acid therapy. Nucleic acid is the material of the cell nucleus which contains DNA and RNA, the cellular components which control heredity and the ability of the cell to reproduce itself. These twisted strands of acid in the cells are the governors of all life processes.

By supplying the body, from external sources, with enough viable nucleic acid, as well as the nutrients these acids require to be properly metabolized, Dr Benjamin Frank has been able to demonstrate a reversal of the ageing process. (Nucleic acid therapy, Benjamin Frank MD, Psychological Library, New York, 1974). He used dosages of RNA between 30mg and 300mg together with B vitamins (as described in previous chapters) in therapeutic trials. The first noted benefit was an increase in energy followed by a gradual improvement in tissue status. He maintains that this approach works by increasing the energy available to the cell; by providing the building blocks necessary for the body to assemble RNA, and by improving enzyme function.

It is the provision of viable nucleic acids and the associated nutrients for their metabolism which is the key to the success of this effort. Foods which provide abundant DNA/RNA material include nutritional yeast, mushrooms, green leafy vegetables, sardines, beans, and organ meats. There are also available RNA-DNA tablets which can be taken in doses of 100mg to 300mg daily, indefinitely, together with B vitamins. These should not be taken by people with elevated uric acid levels, however, such as occur in gout.

A report in *The American Journal of Psychiatry* (Vol. 120, No. 320, 1963) entitled 'Effect of RNA on memory defect in the aged' showed that crude RNA preparations have a positive effect on the nervous system and on memory. Subsequent studies using RNA from yeast sources showed similar results. Intake was high in these trials, between 2g and 75g daily.

This may indicate that a better source of RNA material is via injection. A report in *Radiation Research* (Vol. 29, pages 516-22, 1966) showed that animals which were exposed to X-ray irradiation survived longer when injected at the same time with a preparation of yeast-based RNA, three times weekly. Other research *(International Journal of Radiation Biology)*, Vol. 16, pages 201-209, 1969) confirmed that animals' survival rates went from a mere 5 per cent to over 60 per cent after radiation exposure when they had received RNA by injection.

It seems certain, therefore, that some positive and important influence is achieved by RNA or DNA supplementation. Whether oral sources are as effective is debatable, and seems unlikely, but *some* benefits are noted from the oral form of treatment. It is of such importance for the future of the body that any damaged DNA be repaired that such a form of supplementation could be usefully attempted for some months. A source of excellent injectable RNA is given on page 89. This is available from Germany and is called *Regeneresen*. It comes in ampules of 6mg of organ specific ribonucleic acid derived from young animal cells and combined with RNA from yeast. The organs affected will required different forms of RNA and the suppliers will provide as requested, whether this be for bone marrow, thymus gland, connective tissue, spleen, liver or lymph glands.

Obviously this would require the co-operation and agreement of a physician who would administer the material. Information on this is available from the manufacturers in Germany. This course of action is suggested if radiation damage has occurred, and if protein synthesis has been severely affected. No harm could derive, and benefits could be substantial.

Acidophilus

There remains but one other source of radiation protection. This is reported in *Natural Sources* (Timms and Zar, Celestial Arts, California, 1978) which discusses the protective role of yogurt and soured milks on the damage caused by Strontium 90. These foods have a high content of acidophilus bacteria which are protective of the intestinal flora, the vast colony of bacteria that live in our bowels and which help in digesting our food. Since the digestive tract is commonly damaged in radiation exposure, it is logical that everything possible should be done to enhance this delicate ecosystem within us. Acidophilus in high doses is recommended for all those exposed to radiation, and sources of the best forms of powdered acidophilus will be found on page 00. The eating of live yogurt or drinking of acidophilus (soured) milk products is recommended. Doses of acidophilus should depend upon the strength of the particular cultures, and guidance will be found on page 89.

We have looked at many possible sources of aid in the battle against radiation. We should now turn to a final examination of hazards in everyday life which may be misunderstood. We should also briefly examine different hazards which may be presented by non-ionizing radiation. This is coupled with methods of self-monitoring of the environment, and possible methods of normalizing soil contaminated by radioactivity.

7. The Invisible Enemy

We are constantly exposed to radiation, both ionizing and non-ionizing, and the amount to which we are exposed is likely to increase. Nuclear power is undoubtedly going to have to take the burden of supplying energy in the forseeable future. Coal is plentiful, it is true, but the anxieties and real damage resulting from acid rain, which is an almost certain by-product of the burning of fossil fuels such as coal, makes its long term use in energy production unlikely. Oil will decline in supply over the next decades and, until a better technology comes along, nucelar reactors are likely to be called upon to meet the power needs of industrial nations.

Safer reactors will undoubtedly be developed, and indeed are already in existence in prototype forms. These will reduce the dangers of current water-cooled reactors, either by replacing water with gas or altering the way in which water is used as a coolant, or by quite different technology. Radiation contamination of the environment from such reactors will, hopefully, as a result become less of a danger than is the case with current methods of nucelar power generation. However, nuclear weapon testing will continue in all probability, adding to overall background radiation levels.

The everyday hazards of radiation are, though, not necessarily related to such large scale happenings as weapon testing or reactor explosions and leaks. They are far closer to home, as was briefly outlined in Chapter 1.

Some of the avoidable and unavoidable dangers will be

outlined below, but let us recall that the danger to health and life relating to a given radiation contact depends not only on the properties of the substance but on its chemistry. Something such as radioactive Iodine 131, which may wash onto you when walking in the rain (it is water soluble) presents little danger to you, whereas eating food contaminated with this same radioactive substance will ensure that it reaches your thyroid, and thus is capable of doing great harm. The amount of harm which accrues depends upon the size of the dose. There is no safe level, however. Any radiation is too much. When a substance is radioactive its atomic nucleus is disintegrating and it is this which causes the emission of particles (or waves) of ionizing energy. There are a surprising number of sources of such energy.

David Poch, in his book *Radiation Alert* (Doubleday Canada Ltd, 1985), catalogues the major sources of radiation danger in everyday life, and quite a catalogue it is:

Ceramics: Many items of tableware and decorative glassware contain uranium compounds. Some have as high a level as 20 per cent of their content as uranium oxide. This produces high energy gamma and beta radiation which can reach the internal organs of the body through acidic foods on such ceramics leaking out these compounds. The dose of radiation possible from this source is high if used frequently, possibly exceeding the annual radiation limits thought to be acceptable, from all sources. Those glazes most likely to be contaminated in this way are characterized by a bright, shiny, reflective surface, often in orangey-red, beige or yellow. Local health authorities could be asked to test doubtful ceramic tableware.

Cigarettes: We have already looked at this radioactive source. The tobacco leaf is commonly a source of radioactive Lead 210 or Polonium 210. It is thought that this may derive from phosphate-based fertilizers used in tobacco growing, Alpha radiation derives from the radioactive lead and polonium which is itself a decay product of the lead (as is another substance, radioactive Bismuth 210). These decay products are thought to dissolve in the lungs and to be cleared away, however, this is not true of radioactive lead itself, which is insoluble and remains in the lungs for years, or it can migrate to other tissues, emitting radiation all the time.

Optical glass: This is often a source of radioactivity since rare earths, used in the manufacture often contain radioactive thorium or uranium. Radiation from these, in spectacles, would be small but constant, and is thought to relate to cataract development. Plastic lenses are not radioactive.

Camper's lamps: The white mantle found in camping lamps is possessed of thorium, a radioactive substance which gives off highly charged alpha particles. Thorium eventually decays to form Radium 228 which itself becomes Radon 220, all of which produce alpha radiation. Emission is highest soon after the lighting of the lamp and so this should be done outdoors and left for twenty minutes or so before being brought into a confined space. Care is also suggested when changing mantles.

Building Materials: Radon gas, which is a decay product of uranium is found naturally in many rock formations, and is noted in houses built of brick or concrete. Homes thus constructed have 50 per cent more radon contamination than do wood built homes. Unlike other forms of radiation radon contamination seems to do more harm in constant small doses than in large exposures. Phospho-gypsum a building material derived from by-products of the mining for fertilizer of phosphate rock, is highly radioactive and should be avoided. A comparative study of building materials shows that Granite contains 4.7 parts per million (ppm) uranium and 2.0 ppm thorium. Cement contains 3.4 ppm uranium and 5.1 ppm thorium. Manufactured anhydride, a by-product of gypsum, contains 13.7 ppm uranium and 16.1 ppm thorium. By comparison, sandstone contains only 0.45 ppm uranium and 1.7 ppm thorium.

Water deriving from sources which bring it into contact with radioactive rock often carries radon gas, which becomes airborne eventually, when taps are run or showers used. It is then easily inhaled. Water passing through rock and derived from wells, is higher in radon than that from lakes or reservoirs.

Fertilizers: Many sources of fertilizer are radioactive. These include phosphate rock, the source of phosphorus which is used widely in farming and horticulture. This contains uranium and its breakdown products, which finds its way into the end-product. Tobacco is thought to become radioactive via this source.

Smoke detectors: These are commonly found in public buildings, stores, hotels and many private homes. Some forms have an ionization chamber in their construction which would result in the appliance carrying a warning about radioactive material inside it. If airtight this is safe, but, if not, gamma radiation will be emitted. The greatest danger would occur during a fire where exposure to the core material, Americium 241, could occur. Many other fire detectors use different technology, and are no potential radiation risk.

Colour TVs and Video display units: Colour TVs and VDUs may emit X-rays and this is far more likely in older colour TV sets where X-ray emission was measurable. Modern solid state sets have a lower potential for this. Nevertheless sitting close to a colour VDU or TV set is unwise. Remember that children are more sensitive to radiation damage than are adults. Public video game parlours represent a risk to young people inasmuch as some TV screens leak radiation and expose the players and viewers to the effects of this.

Watch dials: Radium is used on luminous dials of watches and clocks and these should be avoided.

Non-ionizing radiation

This is not the major concern of this book, which is aimed at providing information about protection against ionizing, high-energy radioactivity. Low energy, non-ionizing radiation surrounds us from cradle to grave and its effects are quite different from the dangers described, although in some cases the potential for harm is also great. As David Poch, *(Radiation Alert*, Doubleday, 1985) puts it: 'At the dose level we typically experience in the environment (for example from telecommunications) or in the home (from microwave ovens) or in the workplace (from video display terminals) low energy forms of radiation do not result in immediately identifiable damage to the cells of our bodies. The primary concern with doses of low-energy radiation is the possibility of subtle effects on our nervous system and the chemical "communications system" within our bodies, that regulate virtually every bodily function.'

He notes that whilst there may be a connection between low energy radiation and cancer or genetic effects, we do not know enough about this as yet to estimate risks. The form of the radiation appears to be important, i.e. whether pulsed or continuous, with pulsed forms more damaging. We know little about high voltage electricity transmission effects on people living under, or near, transmission lines, apart from repeated reports of increased degrees of ill health. Biological effects on animals and plants have been noted but little is certain about how these effects are taking place.

It is known, from the work of John Ott (*Light, Radiation and You*, Devin-Adair, 1982) that such apparently safe radiation sources as fluorescent light have a health damaging effect. Since these emit (in the main) light which does not correspond with the full spectrum found in natural sunlight, the effect is different from daylight. This is noted in plants (which will not easily bloom in artificial light unless full spectrum is provided) and chickens in broiler houses (where the addition of full spectrum strip lighting dramatically altered their disease rate and laying capacity) and in humans, where children who were hyperactive and displaying aggressive tendencies in school, were turned into calmer beings by the altering of strip lighting in their classes, from conventional to full spectrum.

We know little of our interaction with the multitude of radiation sources, both low and high energy. What are the effects of radiowaves, microwaves, infra-red light, ultra-violet light, visible light (the only radiation we can see) etc? What are the long-term hazards of irradiated foods. What we do know may be summarized thus:

Extremely low frequency radiation (from electric power lines, VDUs etc.) which is non-ionizing radiation. This is a possible carcinogen but the overall health damaging effects are not understood as yet. It appears that people's behaviour is affected by such radiation.

Radio waves. Also non-ionizing, these appear to disrupt physiological processes including the cardiovascular system.

Microwaves, which are also non-ionizing, can at low levels disrupt physiological processes and at high levels raise body temperature and cause cataracts.

Infra-red radiation at high levels raises body temperature.

Visible light can cause eye damage and raise body temperature.

Ultra-violet radiation can cause sunburn, eye damage, skin cancer and behavioural problems in children (including hyperactivity, when full spectrum light is not also available).

Irradiated food is a source of free radical activity.

We also have evidence of the effects of earth radiation in more subtle ways where the so called ley-lines of the earth electromagnetic discharge appear to influence the health of people living above them. Underground streams alter the electromagnetic energy in the overlying land, and health patterns are different in consequence, showing a higher incidence of cancer for example in people living there.

Much remains to be understood regarding the subtle influences of radiation and electromagnetism on the human body. By no means all such influences are harmful. Bones have been made to knit more rapidly when electromagnetic energy is applied to them. Scans of the body using magnetic resonance will prove safer than X-radiation. What we have ascertained is that it will pay dividends to monitor the environment, to alter it accordingly where this seems beneficial and where it is possible, and to take protective measures which are available through nutritional and other means.

Monitoring the environment

One method is to use a radiation detection device. A personal Geiger counter would seem to be a reasonable safeguard, through which local radiation levels may be checked. Many different versions exist which will give information on various ranges of immediate radioactivity. Some have alarms which are preset to warn against high levels. These can be used on good, pets, water, buildings, soil etc. to monitor the current radiation danger. They range in price from under £100 to many hundreds of pounds and, as in all things, you get what you pay for in terms of reliability and accuracy.

Radiation detection monitors for microwave ovens are available and inexpensive. Personal dosimeters are also available. These are commonly used by people working in exposed situations (medical staff in radiotherapy units, for example). The meters are worn on the body like a fountain pen, and indicate how much radiation you have been exposed to. They require recharging in order to reset them periodically. These are not inexpensive but are advisable for those in contact with radioactive materials.

A similar dosimeter is available for ultra-violet exposure to indicate damaging levels of sunlight. These can be modified to take account of skin type, indicating when a maximum degree of solar radiation has been reached. Different types of radiation monitors can offer a degree of early warning of over-exposure potential. It would be unwise, however, to allow anxiety over radiation to so dominate life as to make it an obsessive factor.

If living in an area of a nucelar power plant, periodic monitoring of water, soil and food etc. is a sensible precaution. Soil which has been contaminated by radioactivity presents a problem. Russian efforts to normalize the soil in the Chernobyl area have highlighted the methods currently available. It was suggested by the experts in this endeavour, from the Institute of Botany, Ukranian Academy of Sciences, that they plant lupins in the soil, as this plant absorbs radioactive elements from the earth. The ultimate disposal of the lupins, however, was thought to present another contamination problem, which ruled this method out. More suitable was the idea of irrigating the land with water to which had been added soluble calcium. This calcium would lock onto radioactive material and carry it down to a safe level, below crop roots. This method can be seen to have much in common with the method suggested for humans in Chapter 3, where calcium from dolomite or bone-meal, is used to bind to radioactive materials in the bowel.

A further suggestion of the scientists would be for a combination of ash and lime to be used as fertilizer before turning the topsoil. The radioactive elements would, it is suggested, then stay below the topsoil and would not rise to the surface again.

The problem with all these solutions is that ultimately a degree of contamination would take the place of the water table below the soil, and this could recycle the danger through drinking water or ultimately rainfall. There is patently no easy solution, but the use of calcium and water should at least remove the danger from the soil and allow crops to be grown safely again.

Background radiation is constant and we must not allow attention to every aspect of this to mitigate against our getting on with the primary objective of living life to the full. The overall message of this book is that there are helpful measures which can be taken either to meet specific known dangers of radiation, or to have general protecive effects against the many hidden sources of radiation which affect each of us. There is no suggestion that by nutritional measures alone total protection is available. However, the many trials on animals, and the human experiences, indicate clearly that protection is possible to a very great extent against even large radiation hazards.

Sources Of Nutrients

Free-form amino acids such as glutathione and cysteine.

Cantassium Company
Larkhall Laboratories
225 Putney Bridge Road
London SW15
(Phone: 01 870 0971)

Nature's Best
P O Box 1
Tunbridge Wells
Kent
(Phone: 0892 34143)

York Medical Supplies
4 Museum Street
York
(Phone: 0904 52378)

Pectin and Algin (tablet and powder form) and Algin with Selenium

Cantassium Company
(address as above)

Fine Green Clay

Cantassium Company
(address above)

Pacific Kelp

Nature's Best or Cantassium Company
(addresses as above)

Vitamins, Minerals and Essential Fatty Acids

Health Food Stores and Pharmacies and:

Cantassium Company (for orotates)
Nature's Best
(addresses as above)

G & G Supplies
51 Railway Approach
East Grinstead
West Sussex
(Phone: 0342 23016)

Natural Flow
Burwash Common
East Sussex
(Phone: 0435 882482)

Water-miscible Vitamins A and E (under trade name of 'Aquacelle')

Vitacare Professional
Chancellor Group Ltd
Freepost
Guildford
Surrey
GU2 5BR
(Phone: 0483 505541)

Adaptogens such as Ginseng and Eleutherococcus

Salus-Haus
Fern Reach
Delph Lane
Daresbury
Warrington

Cheshire
(Phone: 0925 74236)

RNA and DNA in tablet form

Cantassium Company and Nature's Best
(addresses as above)

RNA in injectable form ('Regeneresen')

CPW Rahlstedt Ltd
Buchwaldstrasse 67
D-200 Hamburg 73
West Germany

(Monograph entitled 'Regeneresen' by Professor Dyckerhoff available on request)

Royal Jelly

Ortis
7a-9a Church Street
Esher
Surrey

Pollen Extracts

From Health Food Stores. Brand name 'Cernilton' recommended.

Acidophilus

In the super strengths available as Superdophilus from:
G & G Supplies
(address as above)

As Vitaldophilus from:
York Medical Supplies
(address as above)

Quarter to half teaspoon of the powder of either of these sources of acidophilus should be taken in luke-warm water once or twice daily to help repopulate the bowel when radiation exposure has occurred (or after antibiotics).

Yeast-free Vitamin B

Bio-Health Ltd
13 Oakdale Road
London
SW16
(Phone: 01-769 7975)

Summary Of Radiation Protection Methods

First-line defenders such as SOD and Glutathione Peroxidase

Zinc, Copper, Magnesium as Orotates (for SOD – Superoxide Dismutase)

Amino acids Glutathione and mineral Selenium (for Glutathione Peroxidase).

Second-line defenders: Antioxidants and Free Radical Scavengers

Amino acids Glutathione and Cysteine.

Vitamin A and Beta Carotene.

Vitamin C and Bioflavonoids.

Vitamin E and Selenium (these act symbiotically).

Vitamins B_1, B_5, B_6. (Taken together in high strength B-Complex).

Eleutherococcus.

Zinc Orotate.

(*Note*: Vitamins A and E should be in water-miscible form).

Binders and removers of radioactive material

Pectin.

Algin.

Green Clay.

Calcium (plus magnesium for balance in a ratio of 2:1).
Sources of Pectin (apart from tablets) include apples and sunflower seeds.
Sources of Algin (apart from tablets) from seaweed and kelp tablets.
Sources of calcium and magnesium together in bonemeal and dolomite powders or tablets, as well as individually.
Green Clay should be French *Argile sur fine*.

Protectors of cell membrane structure
Essential fatty acids (vitamin F).
Vitamin E.
Bioflavonoids (plus vitamin C).
B-vitamins Choline, Inositol and PABA (taken as part of high strength vitamin B-complex, or individually.

DNA protectors and regenerators
Vitamins A, C and E.
RNA/DNA tablets.
Organ specific RNA in injectable form as Regeneresen.
Edible yeast.

Protectors of intestinal status
Acidophilus in high strength powders (and as live yogurt).
Fine Green Clay.
B-Complex vitamins.

General body protectors, adaptogens etc.
Eleutherococcus (also anti-oxidant).
Ginseng.
Pollen (also protects cell membrane structures and DNA).
Royal Jelly.
Histidine (amino acid).

Foods containing major protective nutrients, as above, include:
Garlic, onions, brassica family (cabbage, broccoli, etc.), green leafy vegetables, yellow or orange coloured vegetables, eggs, oily fish, apples (and other fruits), sunflower/sesame/linseed

and other edible seeds, organ meats and marrow, mushrooms, yeast, seaweed, soured milks and yogurt.

Dosage and frequency note

Dosages of the various nutrients will depend upon conditions and degree of exposure which has taken place, or which is anticipated. Guidelines are given in the text of the book as to quantities. In the main a number of divided doses through the day are preferable to one large dose. One or more nutrient or protective substance from each of the various groups above should be taken, ideally as a minimum anti-radiation damage strategy. Many, such as vitamin E and the bioflavonoids (and vitamin C) have multiple roles and are very important.

INDEX